the
LITTLE
BOOK
of
GAME
CHANGERS

the
LITTLE
BOOK
of
GAME
CHANGERS

50 HEALTHY HABITS FOR MANAGING STRESS & ANXIETY

Jessica Cording
MS, RD, CDN, INHC

VIVA
EDITIONS

Published in the United States by Viva Editions, an imprint of Start Midnight, LLC, 221 River Street, 9th Floor, Hoboken, NJ 07030.

Printed in the United States.
Cover design: Allyson Fields
Cover image: iStock
Text design: Frank Wiedemann
First Edition
10 9 8 7 6 5 4 3 2 1

Trade paper ISBN: 978-1-63228-068-8

E-book ISBN: 978-1-63228-124-1

This book is dedicated to you, Dad. Those dreams where I pick up the phone and hear your voice are my favorites. And you're right—we are so lucky to have Mom. Thanks for the feathers.

TABLE OF CONTENTS

INTRODUCTION

THANK YOU SO much for picking up this book. I'm so glad you're here. If you're frustrated and fed up and feeling like you just want something to go well, you're in luck: in these pages, I share 50 of the tiny tweaks my clients call game changers.

Sure, I could have written another diet book, but does the world *really* need another book telling you what to put in your face? We're bombarded with diet information all day, every day, but we're not offered much support or many resources for how to figure out which advice applies best to *your* unique situation or how to stay on track toward your goals when life inevitably gets busy, stressful, or challenging.

As a dietitian and integrative nutrition health coach, my work is about food. But while creating meal plans, interpreting lab values, and prescribing therapeutic diets are important, once my clients and I dig a little deeper into all the other stuff going on in their lives, we discover that food is just the beginning.

For example, people regularly ask me for meal plans, but the majority of the time, their greater struggle turns out to be sticking to those plans. My clients tell me that they're feeling overwhelmed by what's going on in their personal or work lives or that stress and anxiety keep sending them back to the unhelpful habits that had gotten them off track in the first place. Loneliness creeps up and anxiety hijacks their best intentions.

My real work, therefore, is helping people change their behaviors and establish patterns that will empower them to stay well for the long term.

Over the years, I've come up with dozens of simple, easy-to-implement strategies that have helped my clients achieve their goals. (I've also relied on these strategies in my own life!) And I'm so happy when I receive feedback like:

- "I've never felt so normal about food."
- "That lunch hack was a game changer."
- "This meal-prep thing is a game changer."
- "I love your little hacks."
- "I feel like I can do this—and keep doing it."
- "I had no idea this could be so easy."

I was riding on the subway one cold night in 2017 when the idea hit me: *What if I put together a little book of game changers?* At the time, my father was very ill, I was feeling incredibly overwhelmed, and the last thing on my mind was writing a book. The more I thought about it, though, the more I realized how much all of those tiny changes were helping me, and, more importantly, I realized I wasn't the only one out there struggling with stress and having a hard time finding the approachable resources I wanted.

So I started jotting down all those hacks and game changers, and I thought a lot about my clients' feedback, and what began to emerge was a story about healthy habits to rely on when life gets real and throws you wild stuff that spikes your stress and anxiety levels. The result is the book you're reading now.

The great news is that nothing I describe here is fancy or expensive or hard to implement. These little hacks are small shifts or changes you can make in your everyday life. You can use just a few or you can use them all—my only rule is that you honor your mind, body, and spirit, and check in with yourself along the way about what feels good.

While my primary area of expertise is nutrition, I introduce other techniques into my work to complement those dietary approaches. Sometimes I discuss subjects related to exercise, mental health, and other lifestyle factors, and sometimes that means I refer to other practitioners. For chapters in this book that focus on topics I am not an expert in, I spoke with individuals who do have that experience and insight to share with you.

Unfortunately, I can't make the stress or anxiety-provoking situations themselves go away (though it would be cool if I could, wouldn't it?). But these approachable tools will empower you to confront the crazy in your life with more calm and confidence than you even knew you had.

CHECK YOUR "VITALS"

HAVE YOU EVER just felt . . . off? Or how about more than off? Have you ever felt like you were falling apart, running around trying to be everywhere and do everything and then collapsing into bed at night, only to find yourself wide awake at 3 a.m. with your mind racing?

Have you ever said to yourself, "Once this month/ project/job search/wedding/divorce/[insert other stressful thing] is done I'll get back to the gym and start cooking and relieve my stress with happy thoughts instead of donuts and wine?"

Have you ever just felt so emotionally drained and disconnected that going on a date or having a conversation with your partner felt like trying to communicate with someone on the other side of a very thick glass wall?

If you said yes to any of these, chances are that one or more of the vital signs of your wellness was (or may still be) out of alignment.

"Vital signs" is a term we hear a lot in relation to our health. Vital signs measure the body's basic functions. The main vital signs that health care providers routinely monitor include:

- Body temperature
- Pulse rate
- Respiration
- Blood pressure[1]

Knowing what the normal or recommended ranges are for your age and sex and also having a sense of what your personal baseline is can help you get a sense of whether you're in a good place. Depending on the health care setting, other measurements may be routinely monitored, such as blood glucose levels, electrolyte levels, lab values associated with certain organ systems, height, weight, and so on.

Vital Signs of Well-Being

In this book, we'll talk about another set of vital signs that will help you track your mental, physical, and spiritual well-being. Taking stock of these aspects of your overall wellness will help you identify patterns and imbalances and enable you to come up with realistic solutions to help you feel—and stay—in alignment. Here are a few big ones:

- energy levels and how they change through the day
- what type of physical activity you're engaging in and how often
- amount of sleep you're getting and the quality of that sleep
- what you're eating and how consistent you are with consuming nourishing foods
- struggles with cravings or addictions
- stress levels and contributing factors
- anxiety levels and contributing factors
- how happy you feel

- how connected you feel to others in your life
- the smoothness of your interactions with others

Examining how we cope with stress and anxiety can also tell us a lot. It's hard to make progress toward our goals when we're out of balance or when stress or anxiety is running the show.

When I was a new dietitian, I talked with my clients primarily about food. But food is really only one piece of a big picture of our wellness. As time went on and I began to integrate more health coaching practices into my work, we'd also explore what else was going on in their lives. Client after client would tell me that stressful situations or things that triggered their anxiety had held them back from applying the concepts we discussed. Either they found themselves seeking solace in old coping mechanisms or just felt so overwhelmed that they couldn't think straight, much less find the energy to try new recipes or face a gym or workout class. They'd talk about their lack of willpower, but it wasn't willpower at all.

Stress and anxiety are very similar and may manifest similarly. However, they are two different things. As explained by the Anxiety and Depression Association of America (ADAA), stress is a response to a threat, whereas anxiety is a reaction to stress.[2] While we may not always be consciously aware of the exact source of that stress or anxiety, the more we're able to tune into what we're thinking and feeling and how we respond to what's going on in our life, the better we're able to do something about it.

In the short term, stress can be helpful—it's what enabled our ancestors to, say, outrun a predator that wanted to eat them. It's what helps a person push through a race or deliver a killer presentation despite jet lag. Chronic stress, however, can negatively impact our health. Countless studies have linked chronic stress to physical and mental health ailments. It can impair our immune system; interfere with our sleep, digestion, reproduction, and cognitive function; and undermine our mood. It's also been linked to weight gain and an increase in belly fat.[3]

So while nutrition education is still a main part of my work, I spend just as much time talking about ways to manage our stress and anxiety as they pertain to our daily habits. My system incorporates regular check-ins these vital signs of mental, physical, and spiritual wellness. I help my clients achieve a more balanced, calm relationship with food and exercise as we also focus on mindset, coping skills, and self-care to support their long-term success. Even when our goals are related to very tangible things like food or a very measurable goal like a race time, getting into the right headspace to support that goal is key.

That said, if you're struggling with stress or anxiety to the point where it disrupts your daily function, reach out to a mental health professional for help. We all have our stuff, and we all deserve to feel well. While food and lifestyle changes can make a big difference to our mental health, sometimes we need a little bit of support. Working with a mental health expert who can help you find the right treatment approach can make a world of difference.

EASE

I encourage my clients to keep EASE in mind as a guide for identifying areas where they may need to address imbalances:

Energy
Anxiety
Stress
Emotions

These are important because they factor a lot into other things in our life.

- Energy: Ask yourself, "What's my energy level? What's energizing me right now? What's draining me?"
- Anxiety: Ask yourself, "Do I feel anxious? How often do I feel that way? What makes me anxious? How does it manifest for me? How do I cope with my anxiety?"
- Stress: Ask yourself, "Do I feel stressed? How often do I feel that way? What causes me stress? How does stress manifest for me? Do I have control over those things?"

- Emotions: Ask yourself, "What emotions do I most often feel? What causes me to feel that way? How am I coping with those emotions?"

The Work-Life Balance Pie Chart

The Work-Life Balance Pie Chart is an exercise I do with my clients to help people get a look at their current work-life balance and compare it to what they would like it to be.

Start by drawing "slices" that represent how much time per week you typically spend on activities related to work, life, and leisure. Here's an example:

WORK-LIFE BALANCE PIE CHART EXAMPLE

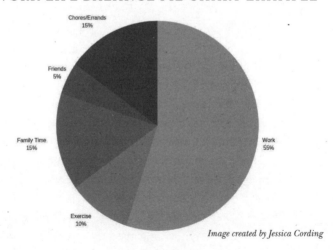

Image created by Jessica Cording

Exactly how many slices are in that chart is completely up to you. For example, if you're dividing your time between a full-time job and a side hustle you ultimately want to grow into your main gig, then maybe you have a few different slices to represent the time you spend on work.

Now divide up another circle into what you wish that balance looked like. Note that this can—and will—change over time, so don't put too much pressure on yourself to write what you think the ideal "should" be. Go with what feels most authentic to the balance you truly want right now. Here's an example:

GOAL WORK-LIFE BALANCE PIE CHART

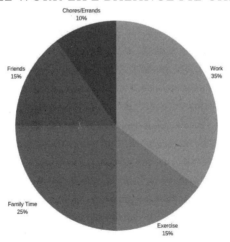

Image created by Jessica Cording

Your reaction to the difference between your current and ideal pies can tell you almost as much as the actual difference itself. In what areas are you spending more or less time than you'd like? Why might that be? What step could you take to change that?

In this book, I'll share the hacks I recommend to my clients and rely on in my own life to address imbalances and support lasting, positive change.

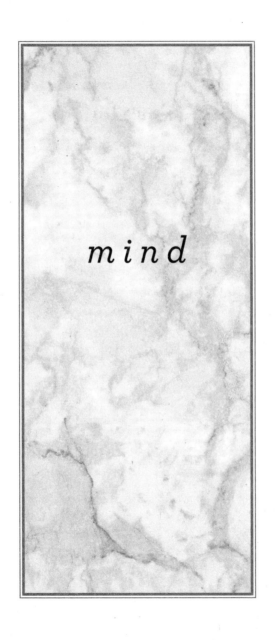

mind

TUNE INTO YOUR INNER VOICE

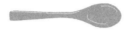

WE ALL HAVE that inner voice that says, "This is what you should do" or "Pay attention to this" or "Don't be an idiot." Sometimes, though, it can be hard to hear that voice amidst the chatter in our brain.

Often, we ignore our gut feelings or we second-guess our instincts either because of our own internal "programming" or because of external pressure to behave in certain ways, make a particular choice, or hold specific beliefs. For example, if you were brought up to act or respond in a certain way, that can color how you behave as an adult, even when those patterns don't serve you. A common one that comes up, for instance, is when we're taught as children to bottle up our emotions, only to find later in life that this can cause us to struggle with things like unhealthy coping mechanisms, such as keeping things to ourselves until we reach a breaking point and have an angry outburst or an all-out meltdown. Or perhaps you have someone in your life who's constantly trying to get you to make logical decisions when you're trying to listen to your intuition?

I've learned this one the hard way a few times in my life, but the story I'll share with you now is one I get asked about a lot—how I came to be a dietitian in the first place.

When I was first living in NYC and working a few part-time PR gigs, I felt totally lost. I'd studied writing in college, but of course writing poems and personal essays wasn't going to pay the bills. I didn't feel like my heart was in teaching writing, I'm a *terrible* waitress, and even though I had my bartending license, no one would take me seriously when they saw how short I was and how young I looked—it would have been like having a twelve-year-old make you a martini. I'd taken a lot of publishing classes in school and had done a marketing internship at a publishing house senior year, so that seemed like the next logical step. Public relations didn't light me up, but I knew that I could learn a lot there.

When I came home at the end of the day, though, I wanted to write. My boyfriend at the time didn't really "approve" of my writing and was critical when I shared it with him. I could have taken his criticism to heart or stopped writing, but I'd already published lots of work under various pen names and had edited several literary magazines in college, and I had a degree in writing—sure, this was my partner, but in my gut I knew that maybe he just didn't speak my language. I stuck to writing when he wasn't around and hiding my folders with my rough drafts so he wouldn't find them. I began to realize, though, it wasn't just a longing to write poems or essays—I wanted to create something that would really help people.

I'd always imagined sharing my work with others or having conversations with them about what was bothering them, finding a way to make them feel better. The problem was, I didn't really know how to make that happen.

My light bulb moment came one day at work when the office manager at a PR firm was showing me what to put in a press kit for a new client. "So you take this bullshit," he said, shoving a bunch of papers into an envelope, "and you put it in this other bullshit," he said, adding a CD to the envelope—we still used CDs back then, that's how long ago this was. "And you make one. Big. Bullshit."

I don't know exactly why that set me off, but I excused myself as quickly as I could and ran into the ladies' room, where I immediately burst into tears. This wasn't the right place for me, but what *was* the right place? What was I actually qualified for? What did I want to do—and not just at that particular moment? What was my *purpose*? I was in full-on ugly-cry mode, shaking, scared, and unsure of what to do next.

I calmed myself down and told myself to dial it back a little. Rather than try to answer those big questions, I thought, maybe I should just think about how I wanted to feel every day, what kind of environment I wanted to show up in.

Sure, there was lots of stuff floating around in my head about what I was "supposed" to want to do (thanks to society, my education, and my impostor syndrome, that sneaky little voice telling me how insignificant and undeserving I was).

5

So I grabbed a pen and paper, tried to tune out the noise, and let the thoughts flow.

What I envisioned was a calm, quiet office with soft lighting. Was it a chiropractor's office? A therapy practice maybe? I went on Craigslist, like I did for pretty much everything back then—jobs, apartments, and dates (everybody read Missed Connections looking for their good story).

And that's how I found the job at the acupuncture practice that eventually inspired me to go back to school to become a dietitian. While I'd been interested in that career path as a teenager, my dislike of chemistry class had thrown me off it. This time around, though, something about working in this practice and studying Chinese medicine in my spare time made me realize I wanted to revisit that old dream.

My boyfriend tried to talk me out of it. I still remember the night I told him I'd applied to nutrition school, thinking he'd be excited for me, but, instead, he was furious that I hadn't talked to him about it first. I guess I had thought that telling him I was checking out programs counted as talking about it? I didn't know I needed permission anyway . . .

I'm still proud of my younger self for not withdrawing my application. It was actually out of character for me at the time—I was so invested in making that relationship work, and I'd already put a lot of myself on hold, but something about this new idea just felt right.

Going back to school and adjusting to a new way of learning was insanely challenging, and I didn't feel like I had any emotional support from my boyfriend, who, through his actions, made me feel that I had to be my own cheerleader. It was a stressful situation: I was crying every day, and my hair was even falling out. There were so many times I was so exhausted and frustrated, I questioned whether I would ever get where I wanted to be, but something in me said to keep going, that things would eventually make sense and fall into place.

Throughout school, I'd thought I had to keep my writing and my nutrition career completely separate. Part of it was that I didn't know any other nutrition students who were writers, and part of it was related to my boyfriend's opinions leading me to believe that nobody in the health care world would take me seriously if they knew I had a creative side.

Then we broke up, and the craziest thing happened.

I realized I wanted some space. I wanted to get centered instead of uproot myself or find someone else to wrap my life around. I was done feeling stressed out and frustrated—there had to be a sane solution.

So I did some math. I calculated exactly how much money I would need to make the rent on a one-bedroom apartment, plus all the utilities. I was about to start my dietetic internship at the hospital, so taking on another part-time job (I already had a couple) wasn't realistic. It dawned on me that I could try my hand at freelancing. I reached out to editors at a bunch of different wellness publications, asking them if they printed student work. A few said no, but a couple were more open-minded and said, "No, but send us your portfolio anyway."

7

Within a few weeks, I'd secured enough writing projects to more than cover that money, and there was no one there to tell me I wasn't allowed to do that.

Whenever people ask me how writing became a part of my nutrition career, I tell that story. In a moment of desperation, I asked myself, "What *can* I do? What do I *like* to do?" All these years later, I'm actually still in touch with a few of the people who took a chance on me back then, and I couldn't be more grateful.

So why am I telling you all this?

In the wellness world, we hear so much about taking care of our gut and nourishing our gut health, but it's just as important to learn how to *trust* our gut and to establish a clear line of communication with our intuition. When we feel like our compass is spinning, it's so much harder to make clearheaded choices that align with our values. Navigating a stressful or anxiety-provoking situation can be so much smoother when we feel clear on what really matters and how to respond in a way that supports the outcome we want, or at least makes us feel more grounded during the process.

Learning how to dial down the background noise and tune into what we need to know is also critical to establishing a more balanced relationship to food and fitness.

Consider the following common situations:

- What type of workout would be best for me today?
- I'm tempted to eat that thing even though I said I wouldn't/I'll feel like crap after—help!

- My sister wants me to do that diet with her and I don't want to but I don't want to say "no."
- Is it okay that I'm eating more than my date?

When my clients are struggling with stress eating or compulsive behaviors regarding food and exercise, we talk about what's going on in their heads so they can become more self-aware and redirect themselves from those unhelpful habits. This also comes up when a client is questioning whether to jump on the same diet or workout bandwagon as a loved one, colleague, or social media influencer they follow.

Having to make decisions can also aggravate those feelings of stress and anxiety that trigger unhealthy coping mechanisms. Feeling unable to make clearheaded choices can become frustrating and exhausting and erode our self-esteem. We'll talk a lot in the gut health chapter about what to feed your gut, but what if you're having trouble hearing what it's telling you?

Here are some of the strategies I use with my clients to help them tune into their inner voice. You can write them out or think them through in your head—whatever works best for you.

Figure Out What Trips Your Wires

We all have those things that, for whatever reason, totally set us off. But instead of getting pissed or upset, get curious! Ask yourself why that particular person, thing, or situation gets to you so much. Don't judge, just see what comes up. This can help you get better at anticipating when you might need to be a little more on top of your self-care (if, say, visiting certain relatives is what does it) or train yourself to take a deep breath when you feel yourself starting to spin into stress mode and tell yourself, "I know what this is. I have the option of dealing with it calmly."

Explore Different Angles

If you're faced with making a decision, a good old-fashioned list of pros and cons works magic. If you're struggling with something more along the lines of an impostor syndrome meltdown, looking for evidence to the contrary will remind you that you're awesome. If you're making yourself sick with worry, to get to the heart of whether that worry is founded in actual facts, run down the list of possible scenarios and see how you react. That can give you valuable insight into what you should actually focus on. If you're feeling like you need help with directions, so to speak, consider different options and their respective outcomes and how you'd feel about each of them.

Ask Yourself What You REALLY Need

When stressed or anxious, we autopilot ourselves straight to our usual coping mechanisms without giving ourselves the chance to tune into what we really, truly need. When you catch yourself doing this (and you *will* get better at catching yourself, I promise!), ask yourself, "Will [insert coping mechanism of choice here] really solve this problem?"

Usually the answer is, "No." Okay, so then ask yourself what will? I use this example a lot, but that's because it rings true for so many of us.

Say you're having a stressful day at work and are craving ice cream. Sure, you want it because it tastes good, but dig a little deeper. Many of us associate ice cream with summer vacation, maybe taking a trip to the ice cream shop with our family, or enjoying ice cream with friends at birthday parties and other celebrations. It's something we associate with feeling relaxed and carefree, a feeling we may want to recapture on days when it seems that the demands of our job are crushing our soul. So pick up the phone and reach out to a friend who makes you laugh, or watch some funny animal videos. Take a walk around the block to escape the office vibe. I had a client who would take her bike for a joyride on her lunch break. She's my hero.

Quiet the Actual Noise

Most of us are surrounded by tremendous amounts of noise on a daily basis. As a self-protective measure, we've learned to ignore the noise. But what we may not realize is that, whether we're aware of it or not, all that noise has interfered with our ability to think and to be aware. Setting aside some quiet time can be tremendously helpful in (re)learning how to listen to your own mind and body. Start with five minutes a few times a week. If you need to set a timer, go ahead. I like to do this while I'm eating breakfast or when I need a short break in the afternoon. Jotting down in a journal the

11

thoughts and ideas that come up during your quiet time is a great way to see what's going on inside your head.

EMBRACE ROUTINE

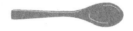

SOMETIMES THE CONCEPT of routine has a negative connotation because it gets lumped in with "the daily grind" or getting stuck in a rut. Or maybe you've heard the term "creature of habit" used to refer to someone who's set in their ways. The word "routine" itself makes some people cringe because it brings to mind visions of a 5 a.m. alarm and a rain-or-shine ten-mile run, followed by a chalky-tasting green smoothie choked down on their commute to work. Of course, that very same image may make someone else jump for joy. Bless them.

However, establishing a routine that helps us take care of those self-care basics that support our wellness is key to staying on track as we work toward goals, and helps us stay grounded in our day-to-day life. Having morning and evening routines, for example, may help provide structure for our day.

The good news is that routines are entirely customizable—and they should be. I see so many people beat themselves up trying to get into a groove with a set of activities that run counter to their natural rhythms and energy: All you night owls who wish you could be morning people, I'm talking to you.

When we ignore our true nature, we're setting ourselves up for failure and frustration, which in turn causes us to doubt our ability to make lasting changes. Yes, you can tweak and adjust, but if you notice that something feels impossible to put into practice or that it makes you absolutely miserable and never seems to get easier, your body and brain may be sending you a message that whatever you're trying to do just isn't right for you—and that's okay.

Here are some tips for getting into a routine. Consider these a jumping-off point to give you some inspiration. And, by the way, it's okay for it to take some time to establish a rhythm. It's also okay to adjust your routines over time to accommodate changes in your life. If, after a certain point, something that once worked for you no longer does, give yourself permission to let it go.

Morning Routines

- Start with a consistent wake-up time. This helps your body get into a regular sleep cycle. Initially this might feel weird, but over time, you'll likely notice that you wake up feeling more energized. You don't have to get out of bed at the exact same time every single day, but keeping it within that same one- or two-hour window (yes, even on weekends) will help train your body to know when it's time to rest and to wake up. If you need to adjust to an earlier wake-up time than you're used to, give yourself a couple weeks, getting up fifteen minutes earlier every few days rather than just suddenly trying to go from waking at, say, 11 a.m. one day to 7 a.m. the next.

- Hydrate. Our cells need water to do all the work they do taking care of us. We wake up dehydrated, so drinking a glass of water first thing can help us perk up like a flower and get ready for the day. It's also great for our skin and helps stimulate digestion to keep things moving regularly. I'm a big fan of lemon water in the morning.

- Move. There's no rule that says you have to exercise in the morning—exercise in general has been associated with improved physical and mental health[4]—but moving in the morning, whether a formal workout, a stretch, or a walk can help get the blood flowing and get your energy up.

- Clear your mind. Whether it's meditation, journaling, writing down your dreams, taking a walk, or enjoying a moment to acknowledge your feelings, a little mental decluttering can go a long way. Think about how much easier it is to get ready when you clear out all the excess stuff from your closet and can actually find the stuff you need. If you're not sure which one of these to start with, I'd recommend journaling. Give yourself five minutes and start by filling in the blank:

Right now, I am thinking _____.

- Fuel up. Tune into what foods and beverages make you feel energized and stable in the morning (for me, that definitely includes coffee!). Make it convenient to include those in your day (i.e., brewing coffee while you get ready in the morning). Stock your home and workspace with your essentials and familiarize yourself with where you can get your on-the-go must-haves.

Bedtime Routines

Having a bedtime routine helps us get the quality rest we need to function. Here are some sleep basics to try:

- Stick to a regular bedtime. I can't stress this one enough. It trains your brain to recognize when it's time to fall asleep. Again, it can be within an hour or two of the desired time.
- Give yourself time to "power down." This one has become something of a cliché, but for good reason. Giving your body and brain some time to shift from "awake-and-doing-stuff" mode to "bedtime" mode can help you drift off with less drama.
- Pay attention to your sleep environment. Make sure the room is cool and dark. Neutralizing any distracting sounds with a white noise machine can help you. Investing in sheets that feel good and choosing colors that soothe you can also go a long

way toward creating a space that feels like a calming oasis, even if you live in a studio apartment.

- Try meditation. If you're not into morning meditations, an evening meditation can be a great way to get into a different mind-set and dial down any loud, disruptive thoughts from the day. Don't think you know how to meditate? Try an app like Headspace, Simple Habit, or Insight Timer, just to name a few.

- When you can't sleep, be gentle with yourself. Rather than tossing and turning and staring at the clock with tears of rage in your eyes (hey, I've been there too), get out of bed and do something mellow. Read, watch TV, knit, clean a drawer—whatever occupies you and redirects your thoughts away from the "why-am-I-up?" loop.

- Choose sleep aids wisely. If you have serious trouble with insomnia, your health care provider can be a good resource for medical and nonmedical approaches and can discuss their validity and safety as well as how to use different ones at different times. I generally recommend trying natural approaches first before turning to prescription sleep medications. For example, I often start by recommending aromatherapy to my clients (more on that later) and discussing overall sleep hygiene with them, such as making sure their sleeping area is cool, quiet, and dark. Melatonin supplements work by increasing levels of melatonin, a hormone that regulates the circadian rhythm (translation: helps signal to your body that it's time to go to sleep). They have minimal side effects and tend not to be habit-forming. However, they won't usually knock you out and aren't meant to be an everyday thing, but when you're traveling across time zones or having trouble getting into a consistent sleep cycle, it can be helpful in regulating your circadian rhythm so that after a week or so, you no longer need the supplement. CBD (the chemical in cannabis that doesn't get you high) is also being looked at for its potential effect on sleep. While prescription and over-the-counter medications are available, familiarize yourself with the risks and have a conversation with your doctor about whether they're safe for you.

Rut vs. Routine

All that said, sometimes it's possible to become too set in our routine and to get to a point where what was once helpful actually becomes harmful.

Here are a few signs that you're being too rigid:

- You cancel plans with friends or avoid situations you would normally enjoy because you don't want it to interfere with your routine.
- You get mad at or "punish" yourself for skipping parts of your routine.
- When unexpected things come up and disrupt your routine, you find it incredibly difficult to cope.

Bottom Line

Embracing a morning and bedtime routine can help you stay grounded and on track. Give it a shot. Take into account your schedule along with your natural energy ebbs and flows. Sure, there may be some trial and error, but once you have a few consistent habits in place (seriously, it doesn't have to be elaborate), you'll likely notice a big difference in how prepared you feel at the beginning of each day and how much easier it is to unplug at the end.

SCHEDULE
YOURSELF IN

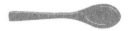

MANY OF US use a calendar to keep track of appointments, deadlines, tasks, and other things we need to remember and make time for. Whether you're the only one in charge of what gets put on that calendar or there are others booking time on your behalf, isn't it amazing how easy it is to give an entire day to other people, only to wind up feeling like you have no time for yourself?

Occasionally, of course, losing control of your own schedule is unavoidable. But when it becomes the norm, it can take a serious toll on your health and well-being. When we don't get any time to recharge, we can begin to feel overwhelmed, stressed out, and anxious about how and when (and whether) everything will fit into place. It can also make us physically exhausted, which can lead to even more bad news for our mental health and impair our cognitive function and immune system. And since lack of time often makes it harder to exercise and make healthy food choices, some may find that their weight creeps up. For others, it can be the opposite, as they feel too exhausted or wired to eat normally.

I went through this myself when I was in my late twenties and juggling seven different jobs. Between shifts at the hospital, corporate wellness gigs, private clients, freelance writing, and other projects, I lived in a perpetual state of exhaustion. I was always the first person to leave a party, and even though I tried to get to bed early to make that 5 a.m. alarm less painful, I'd often find myself wide awake at 3 a.m., heart and mind racing. I barely saw my family or friends. And dating? I tried, but found myself mostly connecting with other burnt-out souls. Bonding over how little time you have for each other sounds cute on paper, but in actual real life? Not so much.

I finally got the message that things had to change during a yoga class I dragged myself to after a tough day at the hospital. I thought I was practicing good self-care, but in all honesty, I probably should have gone home for a nap instead. I'm still not exactly sure how it was possible, but I actually fell asleep in Downward Dog position. Yep, I fell flat on my face, which was exactly the wake-up call I needed. No pun intended.

I finally took an honest look at where my time was going each week, and I realized that nowhere on my calendar had I left any room for myself. I began weeding out nonessentials and delegating what I could. This process can be hard, I know—sometimes it feels like everything is essential or that we absolutely have to do it all ourselves, which usually means we need to dig deeper into our thoughts, feelings, and beliefs to see whether there are some untrue stories we've been telling ourselves. In my case, I started calling myself out on a belief that I had to do every work task myself and say yes to every opportunity without checking in with myself about whether it served the big picture because I was young and single and still early in my career.

To my surprise, all that weeding and delegating didn't solve the problem. Somehow, I still managed to fill my days with things that drained me, and I still found myself falling into bed every night with every muscle in my body sighing. I was physically, emotionally, and mentally drained and starting to wonder whether this was what life was supposed to be like or whether I was just being a wuss. Much-needed reality checks from family, friends, and colleagues reminded me that, no, exhaustion is *not* what life is about.

What finally helped me turn the corner? When I started using a calendar service that allowed people to book meetings with me, it finally dawned on me that I could block off time for myself. Duh. I made sure to set my "opening" and "closing" hours to give myself enough "me" time in the morning and evening, and I started entering my workouts as appointments in my calendar. I also learned to schedule time to actually *get* to Monday-night therapy.

Taking it a step further and scheduling breaks by writing "Jess" on the calendar was the real game changer, though. Seeing my own name on my daily schedule was a powerful reminder that—oh yeah—I mattered just as much as those other things I considered priorities. I would never think of blowing off a client because something "more important" came up, so why was I doing that to myself?

Not surprisingly, I found that investing time and energy in my own health and well-being helped me show up as the person I wanted and needed to be for the people in my personal and professional life. Because I was taking time to recharge my own batteries, I had more energy to give to others.

You don't have to use the exact method I did, of course. There are all manner of electronic and nonelectronic ways of keeping a schedule—paper planners, electronic calendars, apps, and Google docs, just to name a few. Set up a system that suits your lifestyle and needs. And if you have someone else who books your appointments for you, make sure he or she knows your boundaries. If you find yourself feeling guilty at first, think about it this way: investing in yourself will benefit others around you.

One important caveat: even if you're the kind of person who keeps track of everything in your head, I strongly encourage you to keep a written calendar (even if it's digital) anyway. Your own well-being is as essential as any other priority on your to-do list. And there's something about the process of writing down your personal time—and then seeing it on the calendar—that emphasizes the fact that yes, you matter, and increases the likelihood that you'll keep those "appointments" with yourself.

You can write in your own name, you can write "break," you can write the specific activity that you're using that time for. For example, that could be meditation, a workout, or a call with someone who inspires you; whatever works for you and reinforces that the time is valuable.

If rules are helpful, here's a good one to commit to memory: if it doesn't get put on your calendar, it won't get done. Just think of how easy it is to forget things we don't write down. Skeptical? Totally been there. But try it for a month. I'm betting that you'll see some kind of shift.

WHAT HOLDS YOU BACK? IDENTIFY YOUR BARRIERS.

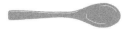

YOU KNOW THAT old saying, "Awareness is the first step"? Well, it's true. One of the most important steps to reaching a goal is identifying the barriers that get in our way. While it can be uncomfortable, get really real with yourself about what trips you up and triggers you in your life. We all have barriers, and that is 100 percent okay.

Think about those times you've veered off from a plan or a promise you'd made to yourself about something you would or wouldn't do. What diverts you? Here are a few common ones:

- Travel
- A stressful day or event
- Unexpected schedule changes or an unpredictable schedule
- Birthdays, weddings, and other celebrations or events with a lot of less-than-healthy foods and beverages
- An emotionally upsetting conversation
- Bad news

- Feeling overwhelmed by events in your life
- Illness and injuries
- A looming deadline you're trying to avoid
- Relationship problems (or lack thereof—aka feeling like you're the only single person alive)
- Loneliness
- Visual cues and external cues to eat, drink, shop, etc.

Identifying our barriers helps us set up a plan to deal with them. A plan, in turn, provides structure and guidance and helps you feel less overwhelmed. Once you're aware of those things that throw you off, a plan acts as a jumping-off point for fixing that behavior.

For example, if you can't ever seem to walk away without a pastry at the café where you pick up your coffee (you've tried having breakfast first—it makes no difference), you can try getting your coffee somewhere else or making your own so you won't feel so tempted. Similarly, if you pass a certain shop or bakery on your usual route and find it hard not to go in there, try going a different way so you don't pass those spots.

If meeting friends for a drink leads to way more drinks than planned (again), tune into what keeps you saying yes to refills. Is it habit? Is it because everyone else is drinking that much and you're worried they'll start asking questions or give you a hard time about it? Acknowledging where your tendency to drink too much stems from arms you with the information you need to shift that behavior.

If drinking one alcoholic beverage after another is just an old habit, start alternating with water or seltzer to pace yourself and avoid getting dehydrated. Nonalcoholic beer and virgin drinks are an option too, but keep in mind they'll still contribute extra calories to your day, so be mindful of how that's fitting into your plans. If real or imagined peer pressure is your downfall, check in with yourself about which it is. Nine times out of ten, people will barely notice you're drinking less. I've even had clients tell me that when friends did notice, they were actually relieved because they wanted to start drinking less too.

If you keep drinking because you associate that with bonding, you may be caught in a loop of thinking that you have to keep drinking alcohol to prolong the experience. Remind yourself that it doesn't matter if you're drinking alcohol or not—it's about that experience of spending time with your friends. You can also try reminding yourself that you'll feel better and remember the event more clearly if you keep your intake more moderate.

The feeling of wanting to belong can lead us to make other choices that may undermine our goals, such as overeating, spending too much money, or joining in a group's negative self-talk. If you've ever been around a table of people talking about how "bad" they're eating or how fat they are or have been, or if you've been in a dressing room with friends or relatives talking smack about their own bodies and found yourself compelled to throw in a self-deprecating comment, you know what I'm talking about.

If travel or a busy or unpredictable schedule throws you off your healthy eating game, then take steps to stay on track with a nourishing diet by making it convenient to eat well. For example, you can stock your freezer with frozen produce and keep healthy staples on hand like beans, whole grains, and canned tomatoes. You can also have groceries delivered when you return from trips so you don't fall into the trap of continuing to eat oversized portions of restaurant food that's more indulgent (and more expensive!) than you'd like because you come home to an empty kitchen.

If shopping is your "thing," I feel you. I'm *extremely* susceptible to emails announcing sales on Old Navy active-wear, particularly when I'm getting tired while working, feeling down, or in need of some escape because I don't want to focus on something unpleasant.

My impulse is to immediately fill an online shopping cart with stuff I (usually) don't need. Or I'll go to a store for one thing I do need and come up with about ten other things I suddenly discovered that I can't live without. When my dad was in the hospital, I spent a huge amount of time in the ICU waiting area, working on my laptop, but also, yes, shopping. And it's rarely expensive stuff! So when my clients get down on themselves for seeking solace in the vending machine, I totally get it, even if my struggle isn't exactly the same. I look at those twelve-dollar sports bras as the emotional equivalent of a pack of M&Ms.

In my case, what helps me keep the habit in check is unsubscribing from those enticing emails (either one by one or using a service like unroll.me) and taking a break from the screen when I feel the urge to shop. That might be a walk around the block, or filling the screen with something else like an online yoga, Pilates, or barre class.

Another thing that comes up a lot for many of us is spending energy on tasks that don't serve the big picture for us. Ever lost an hour to scrolling on social media, only to wind up feeling behind on your to-do list and despairing that your life isn't nearly as fabulous as xyz person you're suddenly comparing yourself to? Social media time can chip away at our self-esteem and derail us from accomplishing the goals we set out to accomplish on any given day. That energy-sucking effect can trickle into other areas of our life, impacting our focus, productivity, and relationships.

If that's you, when you find yourself reaching for your phone, train yourself to ask why you're opening that app. If you need to, set a timer to remind yourself to log off before you go too far down the rabbit hole. Tools that allow you to track your screen time can also be helpful for getting a handle on where your time goes.

Whatever your individual barriers are, don't waste time feeling ashamed. Give yourself permission to be human and set yourself up for success by coming up with a plan to get through those tough spots.

THE POWER
OF INTENTION

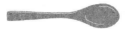

WHEN I WALKED into the reception area of shared work-space, Primary, to interview CEO and cofounder Lisa Skye Hain, the first thing I noticed was the energizing yet calming scent in the air—citrus? (It turned out to be lemongrass.) There were lots of plants, and the lighting was bright without being intrusive. In short, it was unlike any coworking space I'd stepped foot in before. In addition to a beautiful environment with lots of greenery and relaxing imagery, Primary, whose motto is "You work best when you feel great," also offers on-site fitness, yoga, and meditation classes, as well as healthy food and beverage options in the cafe. Clearly, a lot of thought and consideration had gone into each element and how it could enhance members' and visitors' experiences.

Appropriately, my conversation with Skye Hain that afternoon was about the connection between our health and our work performance, but on a deeper level, it was about the power of putting intention behind our thoughts and actions to help us move forward in a positive direction.

When we feel most powerless and ineffective is often

when we feel that life is happening to us, as opposed to us being in control of it. During those times, we feel that we're constantly on defense, reacting and responding to external factors, and shaping our daily routines—and on a deeper level, our habits and big-picture goals—based on outside influences.

Take, for example, staying in a job you hate rather than considering what you could do to improve your situation. Staying put is passive and will make you feel like a victim. That, in turn, could lead to depression and all sorts of negative (and possibly self-destructive) behaviors. A healthier approach is to be intentional, which might mean addressing the factors that make your work environment stressful or toxic, starting to look for a new job that aligns with your core values, or taking steps toward developing a side hustle.

Being intentional in how we approach our day and our self-care can help make us feel more grounded and keep us from turning to unhealthy coping mechanisms when we get stressed out or anxious. Here are some ways to harness the power of intention in your daily life.

Make Declarations

I've always been a big believer that if you want something to show up in your life, you need to put it out there—if you want something, make it known. In those moments when it feels scary to state an intention that feels far away or uncertain, I find reassurance in past examples of when that approach has worked for me, and I draw inspiration from stories of other people who have put that power to use. Before launching Primary, Skye Hain was WeWork's founding Head of Community, where she oversaw operations for their first 275 offices. How she got started at WeWork is an interesting and inspiring story. She had been working in real estate and had decided that she wanted to move on.

She explains, "I said, 'I'm going to use the power of intention and make a declaration to my community and the world and, so to speak, the universe. I am going to make something possible for myself, and I don't know what I'm going to do next, but I'm going to declare it and therefore it will be so.' I had no idea what the heck I was going to do next, but I love creating community and bringing people together."

The very next day, she went to a BNI (Business Network International) chapter meeting. After the meeting, she was approached by Adam Neumann, the founder of WeWork, who told her he might need a mortgage. Skye Hain explained that she was leaving real estate but would be happy to refer him to her partner.

"He said, 'What are you going to do?' I said, 'I don't know. I want to find something that really lights me up.' Having lost my father suddenly in 2004, I'm privy to the fact that life can be gone like that, and it is precious, and therefore we do need to make choices every day that get us excited to get out of bed.

"I said, 'I don't know what I want to do next, but I want to do something I love.' And he said, 'Well, I have this building I took down in SOHO, you should come see it. I'm launching this company called WeWork.'"

That same afternoon she went to see the building that became their first location, and two days later, Neumann offered her a job.

"For me, creating community was what I love, and WeWork was the physical iteration of that. I was with them for fourteen months, and when I left, I immediately knew I wanted to launch my own, but the question was, 'How will I be different?'"

Sometimes we get the idea for how to put our intention into action right away, but it can also take time to evolve and crystalize.

For Skye Hain, the aha moment about Primary came when she was in Oregon, where she had temporarily moved to be with her mother, who was having shoulder issues and needed surgery. She had met her now-husband and partner Brian, who was a triathlon coach and endurance athlete "who was all about living healthy and having fun," she explains. "He lives and breathes and oozes information about how to be well in your body and in your life." Her best girlfriend, Elijah Selby, also became a health coach at that time. At thirty-six years old, Skye Hain says, she began reading ingredients lists and practicing more yoga and meditation and thinking more about the role of wellness in the workplace.

She saw big companies starting to offer those resources

for their employees, but then realized there was no shared office space business doing this for small business owners. And so Primary was born.

Schedule Inspiration

We often think of inspiration as something that strikes us from out of nowhere, but we can play a part in putting ourselves in its path and making time for people and practices that uplift us. Self-care plays a big role in helping us be more receptive to inspiration when we come across it.

That can include rituals like taking a hot bath, journaling, a mindfulness practice, or getting together with people who inspire you. Skye Hain recommends scheduling dinner with friends who bring that out in you rather than someone you'll spend the time complaining with or someone who makes you feel bad about yourself. For her, "it's someone who generates with me and for me and lifts me up."

Social media can be tricky, but being intentional about which accounts you follow and how they make you feel can help you have a positive experience, rather than getting sucked into a negative headspace from scrolling. Skye Hain's criteria is "Women I think are doing things that lift people up in the world and in a way where they make it attainable for others to achieve the same. That's who I want to be in the world—inspiration for others—and so I have to keep myself inspired."

Make Wellness a Priority

Saying you'll "work out more" or "get to bed on time" is very different from setting clear guidelines for yourself to make those goals a reality, such as declaring what you will do and how often, or what time you'll start winding down for sleep, or what steps you'll take to create an ideal sleep environment. Another important step is being in tune with the benefit to your personal and professional life, as opposed to just ticking off boxes in the "wellness" category on that list of Things a Functional Adult Should Do.

Skye Hain has found that, "If you are well-slept, well-fed, and well-exercised, so to speak, you should be able to be so you can be focused, make the best choices, be resourceful, and feel like you have the bandwidth to be resilient."

Of course, we all have those times where we just don't feel on our game. Addressing where we're struggling can help us feel more in balance. "When you're not feeling great in your life," says Skye Hain, "ask yourself these simple questions: Am I sleeping well? Am I eating well? Am I exercising?"

You can also dig a little deeper and think about how well your emotional and spiritual needs are being met. How connected do you feel with the people around you? If something's not clicking, ask yourself why that might be and brainstorm a next step in the direction in which you want to move the needle.

For example, when I have a client who feels badly about the fact that she always eats pastries at weekly meetings with her team members at work. We often talk about what she's thinking and feeling in those situations, what the tone of the room is, and so on. Sure, eating the croissant she said she wasn't going to eat is the glaring "symptom," but what's the underlying issue? If she's feeling pressured to eat out of a desire to "fit in," we might discuss some other ways to bond with her colleagues. We might also discuss what tweaks to make elsewhere in her day to make room for that treat so that food guilt doesn't take up valuable space in her mind that she needs for other stuff. In that case, it's about tuning into how to make a choice that best supports emotional wellness.

Also, don't forget to breathe! Sometimes we need to be intentional about this one, as many of us have a tendency to hold our breath when we're tense or anxious. Skye Hain credits her years practicing Bikram yoga for her belief in the importance of breathing, especially in stressful moments. "I'm so tuned into, 'Am I breathing, am I allowing air to go all the way down into my belly to fill my chest or am I holding it tight?' I visualize the breath go into my shoulders and my neck to soften everything. It allows you to experience life from a more fluid standpoint, and that impacts your mind and your experience of life, business, choices, relationships...everything."

Remember: Baby Steps Are Still Steps
In today's world of instant gratification, it's easy to become fixated on the end result and to compare where we are in our journey to others who are where we want to be, forgetting

that everybody had to start somewhere. We turn it into a story about, "Why am I not there yet?" These thoughts can take us out of the present moment and make it harder to acknowledge (and maybe even celebrate) our progress and appreciate the steps we're taking.

Skye Hain shares a favorite analogy Selby shared with her. "When you want to achieve something and you're feeling overwhelmed, it is usually because you're standing on the ground, looking at a ladder and you think you have to jump from the ground to the top of the ladder. Which is impossible—and plus, you'll get hurt! But you don't need to jump to the top of the ladder—you only need to put your foot on the first rung. That's how we get to the top."

Whether you're thinking about a career goal, a relationship milestone, or a wellness-related endeavor, "It's about steps, and baby steps are steps."

"It comes back to mind-set," says Skye Hain. "We're living in a wild world and a wild time right now with this technology and advances and the accessibility of everything...and it's so important to be gentle with ourselves and to just take it one day at a time and say, 'Just for today, I'm going to do my best. I'm going to be around people who inspire me. I'm going to take care of my body.' Taking care of yourself in those small ways eventually adds up to a big, healthy life. It's a daily practice. One day at a time."

SET ASIDE
DAILY WORRY TIME

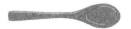

WE ALL WORRY from time to time. However, it's possible for worrying to get out of hand. Aside from being unpleasant, it can be all-consuming and take away mental energy we need for other tasks. It can also seriously dampen our mood and completely disrupt our sleep.

It's hard to drift off into peaceful slumber when our mind is full and those worrisome thoughts are playing like loud music from a party in the apartment upstairs. Even when we do somehow manage to get enough rest, those thoughts can drag us down and make us feel like we're swimming underwater as we're going about our day. Worrying takes a lot of mental energy!

Learn to recognize the difference between critical thinking and nonconstructive, down-the-rabbit-hole-type worrying. For example, having the forethought to look both ways before you cross the street, packing healthy snacks for a road trip where food options may be limited or nonexistent, choosing a complex password, carrying an EpiPen . . . these are all examples of planning ahead for potential problems.

Lying awake at 3 a.m. wondering what to say to that smug coworker if she makes a backhanded compliment about your new haircut tomorrow? Losing sleep worrying about how you're going to afford therapy for your toddler when she's twenty-seven? Rabbit-hole, my friend.

Even when it's a legitimate worry like stressing about how you'd pay rent if you get laid off, fixating on it at the expense of things you really need to focus on in that moment can actually backfire.

To share a personal example, when a hospital I used to work at switched from paper to electronic charting, I was so consumed with worrying about all the negative feedback I was going to get from my supervisor and how it might reflect on my competency, that it short-circuited my thinking and actually caused me to make errors I wouldn't have made otherwise.

A few red flags that may indicate that you're worrying too much:

- Your worries completely consume your thinking and distract you from other tasks
- That problem or stressor doesn't even exist ("yet," you argue)
- You can't actually do anything about that concern
- You get stomach pains, notice changes in your heart rate, start clenching your jaw, or experience related tension headaches when you worry

While it's totally normal for worries to occasionally bubble to the surface, it's important to remember that you *can* change your response. Start by asking yourself, "Is this thing a priority right this minute?" Most of the time, it's not, so here's what to do with those worries: Set aside daily worry time. You can be as loose or as structured about this as you like. Some people prefer to sit in a quiet place (soothing cup of tea optional) or even lie down. Others might find it useful to do it while you're doing something somewhat active like taking a walk or cleaning or folding laundry. You could also journal out your worries in a notebook—it can help you feel like you're really "getting it out" and that you can (literally) close the book on it and walk away after.

Whatever approach you choose, put fifteen minutes on your calendar, set an alert on your phone, or simply just make a point of setting aside a few minutes each day to let your mind go to town on the worrying. The only catch? Once that time is up, you move on with your life.

After your worry time is up, when you start to feel a worry rising, remind yourself that you can return to that thought when it's time to worry. This might feel weird at first, but over time, it can make a huge difference in the amount of time and energy you spend worrying. I know this sounds hard, but I promise it gets easier with time.

TAKE A TECH BREAK.
SERIOUSLY.

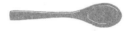

TAKING A BREAK from technology can be damn near impossible. I know I've certainly rolled my eyes when someone has talked about how leaving their phone at home changed their business or how they don't respond to emails on weekends because they're completely present with their adorable family. The idea of a silent retreat or even just a wedding where cell phones are banned makes me really anxious. I'm legitimately proud of myself for remembering to turn my phone to Do Not Disturb when I'm at an event.

The struggle is real. For someone whose work involves electronic contact with clients and lots of screen time working on things like writing, research, and social media, it can be hard to unplug. I was once invited to a wellness retreat that was geared toward "unplugging," and yet in the contract was a list of required hashtags to use when posting to social media about my experience.

Ever heard the term "appsturbation?" Yep, it's that thing where you're in bed with your phone going to town checking apps. All those little micro-hits of the feel-good brain chemical dopamine feel pretty awesome in the moment, but before you know it, an hour has passed. Or three.

Of course, this doesn't just happen in bed at night—we're on our devices all day, every day. We're also surrounded by screens, speakers, and other technology sending us signals and vying for our attention. Maybe you've experienced that phenomenon where you unlock your phone to look something up or jot something down, only to get sucked in to a notification from another app and then completely forget why you'd reached for your phone in the first place.

You used to be able to get a break and have an excuse to go MIA on an airplane, but thanks to in-flight Wi-Fi (which, let's be real, has its perks when you're on a writing deadline or want to stream a movie to pass the time), that's no longer the case. Wi-Fi on public transportation is even a thing now.

Don't get me wrong—technology serves a purpose. GPS in your car, for example, can be super helpful when traveling to somewhere unfamiliar. Social media can help us build our networks and stay connected to people who live and work far away. And, chances are, you probably know at least one couple who met online or via a dating app.

However, as I'm sure you're well aware, excessive screen time can be harmful to our physical and mental health. Technology can distract us and make us feel like we're being constantly interrupted, thanks to frequent notifications. Social media can also be a major trigger for stress and anxiety, especially if current events or "compare-itis" that flares up when you're scrolling sets you off. This lack of focus and subtle sense of feeling less-than-awesome can trickle into other areas of your life and significantly disrupt your day and interactions with others. Not sure how much time you're spending in front of a screen each day? There are actually apps that log every second so you can see exactly how much of your day you're spending online and what you're spending it on. The idea is to use those insights to come up with ways to change your habits.

Taking a little tech break as a regular part of your day or week can help you avoid that overloaded feeling.

Here are a few simple ways to take a temporary break from technology:

- Set aside time to put your phone in "Do Not Disturb" mode or at least turn the ringer off. When you're sleeping or in a workout class or at a movie, those are some great times to unplug. But it's also a great idea for situations where you want to be especially focused, such as a meeting, when you're out with friends, or at an event where you don't want to be distracted. Worried about missing something important? Most phones let you set "favorites," whose messages will still get through to you.
- Set timers during your workday to remind yourself to get up from your computer and stretch, take a walk around the floor, or go do another non-tech task.

- Disable nonessential push notifications on your phone.
- Put your phone in a drawer while you're working if you know you can't *not* look at it.
- Set "office hours" for yourself (no matter where you work from) to set boundaries for checking and responding to emails and messages.
- When you're out with friends or colleagues, unless you're waiting for an important message, keep your phone *off* the table.
- Set yourself a "bedtime alarm" to remind yourself to power down for the day. Do not fall into the "one-last-thing" trap. The truth is that 99 percent of those last things can just as easily wait until tomorrow.
- Get a real alarm clock and keep your phone out of your bedroom. At the very least, keep it out of arm's reach.
- Turn off the TV, music, podcast, and other sources of noise in your home or workspace for at least a few minutes each day to give yourself a chance to enjoy the silence. If you have a journaling or meditation practice, this would be a great time for that.
- Instead of scheduling a phone call, meet friends or colleagues for a walk to catch up or talk shop.

These are just a few of the many ways you can reduce your use of technology in your day. Being aware of where you struggle most will be a good starting place in figuring out which one to try.

Also, if you're not sure you can do it, set a measurable limit. You could try making one of these changes for two weeks and track any changes. Or you could try a month of practicing that change a few days per week. Weekends, vacations, and other times you don't need to be as worried about being on time or plugged in can be a great time to experiment as well.

For example, if the idea of trying a new wake-up system on a weekday freaks you out because you're worried you'll be late, start using that old-fashioned alarm clock on weekends or nonwork days and keep your phone out of the bedroom. You might find it easier to make it an everyday thing if you give yourself time and space to test it out.

REMIND YOURSELF OF
WHAT'S GOING WELL

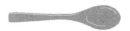

SOMETIMES WHEN I'M walking or doing yoga, I'll talk to whatever you want to call it: a higher power, God, the powers that be—sometimes I talk to my dad. I remember this one night in particular, I kept saying, "I really want to have a positive experience." It was in regard to a specific situation in my life at the time, but honestly, that little prayer-like statement could have applied to a lot of things that were making me feel overwhelmed.

I don't necessarily go into these "conversations" expecting an answer or response, but this particular night, I heard it loud and clear as I settled into Savasana ("corpse pose," which is typically done at the very end of a yoga practice). "You want to have a positive experience? Then *let* yourself have a positive experience."

"Oh, duh. Thanks."

It's so easy to get caught in a loop listing all of the things we're failing at and screwing up, or all the things that are going wrong in our world. There's tremendous power, though, in reminding yourself of what's going well.

Research has shown an association between positive thinking and our physical health.[5] Using brain imaging, researchers have actually been able to observe that positive emotions can trigger "reward" pathways in the brain and that the longer those positive feelings last, the longer the activation of those pathways lasts, helping that person experience a prolonged sense of well-being. Pretty cool, right? Hearing "think positive" from your mother or your best friend is one thing, but seeing on a brain scan that positive thinking makes a difference takes it to a whole new level.

When we're constantly focused on what we need to change or on what we're doing poorly, that negative self-talk can trickle into other areas of our life and drag us down. I know it can be tricky to reframe a crummy situation into something positive. Some of us also come from families or social circles where complaining is how we communicate. Others have been trained to think that it's bad to let on that we like ourselves or are proud of our accomplishments, so we automatically dial down the joy. But if we keep priming ourselves to fail, that's exactly what will most likely happen.

The Power of Positivity

Replacing negative, anxiety-provoking thoughts with positive ones (whether those positive thoughts are related to the original thought or not) has been associated with a reduction in worry.[6] So yeah, maybe you're sweating a deadline or beating up on yourself for eating the cookies you swore you'd avoid, but spend a few minutes thinking about how well you handled a tricky conversation at work, or the delicious, healthy lunch you made.

Why is this helpful? Making a habit of noticing the positive can retrain your brain to more easily recognize the choices that make you feel well and stable so you can make more of those choices. Making this a regular practice can also help you become more resilient over time, so that when troubling things come up—as they always do—you can gather your energy and deal with those stressors more effectively than you might have if you'd gotten sucked into a negative thought pattern.

If saying nice things to yourself feels super weird, you're not alone. I know that when I first started making gratitude journaling and affirmations a part of my day, I felt really uncomfortable. I felt like the second I wrote down something I was proud of, someone was going to swoop in and shake a finger at me for daring to think I deserved to feel good about myself.

I'll admit that even now sometimes there are days when I have to remind myself of the power of noting what's going well and what I appreciate myself for. One time that stands out for me is the week my dad died. He went into the hospital on a Saturday morning with complications from his pancreatic cancer, and on Tuesday night, he passed away. The days in between are a blur.

As someone who had worked in hospitals for years, it was hard to be on the other side of things, watching what was happening but being unable to do anything. Each morning and evening, I actually wrote in my journal that I felt kind of stupid even bothering to try thinking of positives, and yet I continued to show up for myself. I kept it simple: "I now allow myself to feel love and to feel grateful for my family."

Even in those last days, my dad kept up his sense of humor and upbeat attitude. He was more concerned about the rest of us, asking if we were okay, if all the monitors and the alarms scared us. And of course I will never forget the morning he had a heart attack and just *had* to let the rapid response team know that I was single.

"How could I be in a room full of hot doctors and *not* mention it?" he later said. We teased him mercilessly. Even though it was one of the worst days of my life, I still can't help but smile when I think of that part of it.

So that night I wrote that I appreciated myself for laughing, for seeing the love in that moment instead of being embarrassed. That little bit of lightness helped cut through the heavy dark.

Try It

If acknowledging good things makes you squirm, you can start small. If rolling your eyes makes it easier, go for it. Here are a few easy ways to get into the habit of reminding yourself of what's going well:

- Daily affirmations. You can start with something simple, like writing, "I deserve to be happy" each morning.

- A gratitude journaling practice can be incredibly powerful. Each night, list a few things—tiny (delicious coffee) or huge (landed a promotion you've been working really hard toward)—that you're grateful for.
- Do a nightly check-in with yourself about what you did that day. What's one thing you're proud of or feel good about? Even little things like drinking enough water, paying your phone bill, or not spacing out in a meeting count!

It might feel weird at first, but after a few weeks, you may notice that you're talking to yourself differently, with a more encouraging tone.

KEEP A MONEY JOURNAL

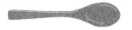

MONEY IS A major source of stress and anxiety. If it's not about not having enough, it's about not knowing what to do with what we do have. It's about all the emotional hang-ups and triggers we have when it comes to money, many of which were learned as kids.

According to a 2017 report by the American Psychological Association, 62 percent of respondents noted money as a source of stress.[7] Fear of the unknown, or generalized anxiety about whether we'll have or make enough, can hijack our thoughts and may even block us from making money. Because we're so fixated on it, we may actually miss opportunities to make sound money choices because we're distracted by too many negative thoughts or anxieties.

Planning and tracking can help dial down the money drama by arming us with data we can use to make necessary changes to support our goals. I spoke with Ashley Feinstein Gerstley, aka The Fiscal Femme, a money coach and author of *The 30-Day Money Cleanse*, whose mission is to demystify the world of money and personal finance to help people get a handle on their money struggles so they can enjoy their life fully.

Money—and our messed-up relationship with it—is a major contributor to stress and anxiety, she explains, and we often feel that we're alone in feeling a lack of abundance and organization in the financial aspect of our health. "In a lot of ways we're not set up for success. There's missing education, [and] in our society we don't talk about money. We deal with it every day but we don't talk about it openly."

It's also an emotionally charged subject, she adds. "We tie up our net worth and our self-worth." So when you're not feeling great about money, it can trickle into how you feel about yourself overall. There's also a lot of shame connected with money, whether that be shame over not having enough, or shame related to having money if you grew up associating money with greed. The latter can make it hard to make or hold on to money because you're unconsciously blocking yourself, she says.

Feinstein Gerstley often has her clients keep a money journal. "A money journal is where you track what you spend, what the item costs, and your emotions around that transaction. It sounds very simple, but we're not usually conscious of where our money's going, and magical things happen when we become aware of that." Seeing what we're doing, she says, can help us let go of the negative habits that hold us back. "Everybody gets different insights from it."

An example she often shares is, "We'll say we can't afford a vacation," and yet when we do the money journal, "we find out we're spending $1,200 a year on small everyday expenses we don't even think about or even really enjoy, like tea or coffee."

How to Keep a Money Journal

You can use a notebook, the Notes section in your phone, an Excel spreadsheet, or an app to track where your money goes. Write down the amount, what you spent the money on, and, after you get good at it, if it's helpful, the emotions you had before and after the purchase or transaction. Aside from cluing you in to how much you spend in different categories, keeping a money journal can also show you any patterns you may have with emotional spending, or highlight areas where you may need to spend more—or find ways to cut back.

This is especially great if you work for yourself or aspire to leave your current job and start your own business. Take it from someone who once wondered whether I was truly "ready" to strike out on my own. My money journal reassured me that I would, in fact, be able to pay my bills, and that knowledge allowed me to proceed calmly—or at least more calmly than if I'd just jumped in without knowing how big the net was.

You may also want to track what you earn in a separate place. Similarly to how reminding yourself of what is going well in your life can work magic on your mind-set, seeing those numbers rise can help you get into a more abundant and receiving frame of mind.

If this sounds tedious, try it for a month. If you can't stand the exercise, give yourself permission to give up, but

I'm confident that you'll learn some valuable information about yourself and your money habits. Also, knowing you have to document every purchase can help you be more mindful about what you spend your money on. The big-picture payoff? Fewer money worries waking you up in the middle of the night.

Then What?

Seeing what your spending patterns look like can actually help reduce the drama around money in a big way. Feinstein Gerstley sees this with clients all the time. "Each experience shared with me has brought the individual to the same conclusion: it's actually less scary when it's out on paper and you can do something about it."

The insights you glean from your money journal will enable you to put together a plan for moving forward. Break down your goals to make them more manageable, Feinstein Gerstley says. For example, if your journal reveals that you're spending a ridiculous amount of money on coffee, your knee-jerk reaction might be to vow that you'll never spend another dime on coffee again. Instead, try something a little less ambitious, like "Today, I'm *not* going to buy coffee, and I'll see how it feels." You can decide to make your own at home, make do with the office coffee, or skip it altogether.

If you're working on another goal in your life, such as improving your physical health, it may also be helpful to check in with yourself about what your spending should look like in that area. "I hear a lot, 'Oh, I want to eat healthy and that's going to be so expensive.' It's an excuse we make—'Because I'm being healthy, I need this expensive product'—when you might need to look at how much water you're drinking. Don't overlook the cheap stuff that's important for your health!"

"In a lot of ways," she adds, with nurturing your physical and financial health at the same time, "there's such a win-win. Often, when I'm doing better in my money life, my health is looking better. A way to look at it would be aligning our values with our spending. We're being conscious and intentional with the dollars we spend."

REWARD YOURSELF

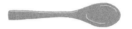

IN MANY WAYS, we've been programmed to think that praise and validation come from external sources (the teacher that gives your grade, the boss who praises you on your hard work, the partner who tells you how great you look), but it can be hard to deal with the reality that sometimes our best efforts go uncelebrated.

And it's not that you're not worth celebrating! People are busy and distracted—or as my mother would say, they've got their head too far up their own ass to even notice what's going on with others. And sometimes, we make something run so smoothly and look so easy that others have no idea how much time and effort went into that finished product or result. Naturally, we feel a little resentful in these moments.

This is why rewarding yourself for completing projects and important tasks is so valuable.

In my coaching practice, I often see people turn to food and beverages as their rewards. Sure, those are easy options, but they can also become unhelpful habits. Have you ever thought something like, "I worked really hard today—I deserve this glass of wine!" The first few times you do that, the wine feels celebratory. But after a while, it simply becomes a nightly goblet that doesn't even feel that special—you just "need" it to make the day feel complete.

Of course, wine is just an example. It could be any food or drink. What's tricky is that when we put food on a pedestal and turn it into a reward, as opposed to something more neutral, we're infusing it with drama and charging it with emotions. It becomes something we have to earn, or something we use to soothe ourselves with when we're not getting the validation we need from other sources, rather than looking within for validation or acknowledging our efforts and accomplishments in meaningful ways.

Rewarding ourselves in other (read: non-food, non-drink) ways, though, can help us feel appreciated, confident, and motivated as we work toward our goals.

Our brain actually has "reward" pathways, and a major one is the mesolimbic dopamine system.[8] In this pathway system, the brain learns to detect pleasurable— aka rewarding—stimuli and motivate the individual to repeat the activity that led to the activation of that pathway. What's more, working with other parts of the brain that control memory and perception of environmental cues, it will send signals telling that person whether a stimulus is rewarding or not. So if you've ever wondered why it's so hard to say, "No thanks," to the chips or chocolate you said you wouldn't have in the office snack drawer, it's not that you lack willpower—it's that your brain is wired to seek pleasurable experiences, something you likely could use at 3 p.m. on a stressful day.

A reward can be something big or something tiny, but it should be something you really want and will feel motivated by. Deciding ahead of time what you want that thing to be will help you keep your eye on the prize, so to speak. It can also make the experiences and purchases you choose as rewards more meaningful and even continue to motivate you in the future.

One of my favorite personal examples is that after getting paid for one of my first big writing projects, I bought (much-needed) new pillows. Even now, laying my head down on them every night is a little reminder of that sense of accomplishment.

Here are a few ways to reward yourself:

- Give yourself a half hour to read, listen to a podcast, or take a walk in the middle of your workday.
- Take a day off.
- Spend time on a restorative hobby that feeds your soul.
- Buy yourself flowers.
- Sleep in—or go to bed early.
- Make yourself a nice meal and sit down and savor it at whatever pace you want, instead of rushing.
- Treat yourself to a massage after a busy week or month.
- Buy a big-ticket item you've been wanting.

- Purchase something that will upgrade your fitness routine like new sneakers or an outfit, a yoga mat, or a package of your favorite class.
- Purchase items to make your living or work space more welcoming.
- Plan a trip you've been dreaming about.

The only "rule" is to reward yourself with things you actually want and that will mean something to you, and not things you *think* you should want.

SAY "NO"

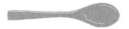

I STILL REMEMBER my "no" aha moment. I was in the coffee line behind another member of a weekly networking group meeting, and I was going down a guilt spiral, listing all the reasons I couldn't help with something she'd asked me to sign up for.

"'No' is a complete sentence," she said. Her tone, though not unkind, implied that my extraneous apologizing and explaining was super annoying.

My jaw dropped. My mind was totally blown. I felt like a babbling rookie, but was so grateful for the reality check.

There are lots of reasons it can be hard to turn down a request or decline an invitation: Maybe you're worried about hurting someone's feelings or are afraid it will reflect negatively on you. Will you seem like you're being selfish or greedy? Will saying no look like a sign of weakness? What if this is someone you hope to work with or get to know better in the future and you're afraid that if you say no once, they'll go away forever?

Saying no and setting boundaries with our time is so

important, though. You probably don't need me to tell you that overloading your schedule with excessive obligations, events, and projects can lead to burnout and resentment. It can also prevent us from actually progressing toward our goals because we get so bogged down in the day-to-day.

If it helps, remind yourself that saying "no" to things that don't serve your big picture leaves room for the things that do serve you. If that's not enough (and I totally get it), here are a few ways to say "no" without feeling like a jerk:

- *Change it into a "not right now."* Say something like, "This sounds great and I would love to be involved, but I can't take this on right now."
- *Thank the asker.* "Thank you" is one of the most powerful phrases in the English language. It takes the edge off and adds a positive note to the conversation. You can keep it simple with something like, "Thank you for taking the time to reach out. This sounds great but I'm not able to do this."
- *Practice.* It sounds cheesy, but you can practice saying no with a friend or even on your own to help you build up the confidence. You can also start by saying no in low-stakes situations. You probably already do and don't even think about it! If you're in a restaurant and someone asks if you want pepper and you say, "No thank you"—use that as evidence that you're capable of saying no.
- *Do your research, if needed.* I know I can say that

we never owe anyone an explanation and that there are things that are nobody's business, but there will always be situations when a one-sentence answer may not be enough. If you suspect that you'll need to follow up with an explanation, have one prepared. You'll feel calmer and avoid stepping backward into a lie or an awkward half-assed story that makes no sense that you regret the second it comes out. It also cuts down on oversharing if you're prone to honesty bombs like yours truly.

- *Be firm.* You're allowed to say no, and once you say it, stand by it. If you start to waver, you might end up feeling even worse than if you'd taken on something that didn't feel right to you.

Own your boundaries and have no shame about your deal-breakers. Some deal-breakers may be more on the "universal" end of the spectrum (working with someone who exhibits mean or abusive behavior), whereas some will be more specific to you (going above 28th Street). Don't be afraid to stand up for what's truly important to you.

VISUALIZE "HAPPY"

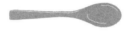

PHOTOGRAPHS CAN BE tremendously impactful in both positive and negative ways. I don't know about you, but I grew up knowing quite a few women who kept photographs of themselves at their thinnest posted on their refrigerator. Curious "tell me why" Sagittarius child that I was, I had to ask.

The conversations often started with something along the lines of, "Who's that lady in the picture?" or "But I thought you hate the beach."

The women would usually explain that the photo was meant to deter them from eating because they were trying to lose weight and look more like they did in that picture on the fridge. I even had one relative who had a decorative cow with a word bubble coming out of its mouth that said, "Holy cow, you're eating again?"

As a young kid, I couldn't wrap my head around why everybody seemed to be on a diet. That changed of course, as I got older and went through the experience of growing up in a culture obsessed with outward appearance where women are (still) trained to view deprivation and restriction as the path to greatness.

I eventually saw that these women were using those photographs as thinspo before #thinspo was a thing, but what I always found interesting was that they never seemed to get to a place where they felt happy with their body, regardless of whether they reached that magic number or clothing size.

Something I started as an experiment with a few clients has since become standard practice for me. Rather than use a picture of yourself where you're at your ideal weight as a motivator to make healthy food and fitness choices, use a photo where you look—and are—happy. Why? That positive energy can spill over into other areas of your life and can support mind and body wellness.

It might not seem like a huge deal, but seeing yourself happy puts you in that headspace, connecting you to the positive energy you felt when you took the photo, and reminding you of those good feelings. Being more connected with those good vibes on a daily basis helps you stick with habits that help foster overall happiness.

Don't believe me? Think about how much harder it is to get out of bed and go to the gym on a day you feel awful about yourself than it is on a day you're feeling upbeat and excited about your life. You don't have to post it on your fridge, but put your "happy" image someplace you'll see it every day and let yourself feel that positive energy. It's a subtle shift, but powerful.

AROMATHERAPY

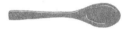

I'VE JOKED THAT when I was first in school studying nutrition, I felt like the freak in the corner talking about aromatherapy. I remember thinking all my classmates were there to learn just the conventional stuff like organic chemistry and medical nutrition therapy, and I felt out of place because I was interested in complementary and alternative treatments. I'd been introduced to the use of essential oils in a volunteer position at an integrative HIV clinic, and even before then, at home, so it made total sense to me that scent impacted mood, energy, and cognitive function. When I was in high school and preparing to take the SATs, for example, my mother gave me a Ziploc full of cotton balls soaked in peppermint oil. "To help you focus," she explained. She instructed me to sniff them while studying and then to bring a similar bag with me on the day of the exam.

So what is aromatherapy, exactly? Aromatherapy is the use of essential oils of flowers, herbs, and trees to enhance your physical, mental, emotional, and spiritual health.[9]

Essential oils are generally used by inhaling them or diluting them and applying them to the skin. Diffusing an oil so the scent can fill a room or space like a car (try it—it's lovely) is a popular way to enjoy aromatherapy. Different oils may be more suited to different applications.

The olfactory (smell) system has been shown to be involved in mood, behavior, and cognitive function.[10] Have you ever been in a cab or in line at a store or in an elevator and found someone's perfume so unbearable you felt anxious and couldn't wait to get out? On the flip side, have you ever walked into someone's home and felt immediately at ease because it smelled pleasant or familiar? Are there certain scents that trigger strong memories or feelings for you? That's your olfactory system at work.

We can use aromatherapy to help shift our mind-set, alleviate stress, and improve our cognitive function, too. I spoke with Ryan Smith, founder of New York City's 5 Point Acupuncture, who uses aromatherapy in his practice as well as in his own self-care routine. "Self-care is where the oils really shine," he said. He finds them especially useful for stress management, promoting restful sleep, supporting healthy digestion, and as a part of a proactive health care routine that assists in reducing toxic load and helping the immune system function optimally.

Here are a few easy ways to start:

- *Lavender* has been shown to be effective for helping ease anxiety, stress, and depression as well as insomnia.[11]
- *Peppermint* oil has been used for treating digestive issues, pain, headaches, and the common cold. If you're someone who's prone to tension headaches, this can be a good one. It's also been shown to help boost memory and cognitive function.[12,13]
- *Grapefruit* and *Lemon* essential oils have both been studied for their potential to boost mood.[14] They each have a nice, cheerful smell that's a good way to brighten a chilly or dark day.
- *Rose* oil has also been studied as a potential mood-booster[15] and has been shown to help promote feelings of relaxation.[16] This is a great one if you're feeling wigged out and overwhelmed.
- *Rosemary* is another great one for promoting focus. Studies have shown it to have a stimulating effect on cognition.[17]

When asked to narrow it down to a top three, Smith recommends lavender, peppermint, and lemon. "Together they provide such a broad base—it's almost like a Swiss Army knife. You've got a central nervous system relaxant, a stimulant, and a detoxifier." Another one he loves and uses frequently is frankincense for fostering a sense of calm, stabilizing mood, and gently relieving fatigue.

Start with a few and see what you respond to. Smith stresses that it really is worth paying more for the good-quality varieties. Start with a few and see what you respond to. He lets his patients smell a bunch of oils, and the one that they become "obsessed with," as he puts it, signals that there is something in that oil they need and are responding to. In my own life, I keep lavender oil on my bedside table to dab on my wrists every night to help me chill out. On days I'm working on a big project and need to focus, I diffuse peppermint or rosemary oil. When I'm sad, grapefruit is my go-to. I use blends with rose in them when I want to feel calmer and happier. A combination of citrus and vanilla are what I turn to when I want to feel more upbeat but calm.

We'll get more into this later, but there are other scents that you can also use as part of a cleansing ritual to clear stale or negative energy. Also know that if essential oils just aren't your thing, you can enjoy similar benefits with scented candles, creams, cleaning supplies, and the like. Tune into what you like and why you like it.

CHANGE YOUR PASSWORDS: THOUGHTS BECOME THINGS

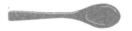

ONE OF THE most valuable things I ever learned was that our thoughts become things. What we put our minds to becomes our reality. Manifesting is a word you may have come across. Maybe you're into it, maybe you're like, "That's a little 'woo' for me," but it's a thing.

The goal is to manifest what we want by focusing on what we desire and taking intentional steps to make those things reality, but it's also possible to manifest what we don't want by becoming overly fixated on them. For example, have you ever been so worried about making a mistake that your hands were shaking or you were distracted and made the exact mistake you were worried about making? Have you ever ordered a "coffee, no cream" and been handed a cup with lots of cream in it because the word "cream" was what came through super clear whereas the word "no" was less emphasized?

When there's something we want to accomplish, we're conditioned to think we need to hustle like crazy to make it happen without giving much attention to the nature of our thoughts and to how we're taking care of ourselves and holding that space for what we want. An example might be working around the clock and letting stress rule our thoughts and actions without questioning where that stress is coming from and what effects it's having on our situation. While it's still beneficial to organize and prepare (think: a business plan for the year ahead, a book outline), doing the inner work on ourselves is when a lot of people see the real magic happen. When I say "inner work," I don't mean anything that far out there—I mean exploring our feelings and beliefs and taking thoughtful steps to shift what needs shifting. Inner work could be journaling, therapy, meditation, mindfulness, or another practice that helps you tune in.

Similarly, what we read and write can also seep into our minds. Have you ever typed something you were saying out loud or vice versa?

It's easy to get distracted from your goals and from the positive thoughts you're trying to nurture, so reminders to redirect your thinking can be so helpful. One of my favorite little hacks is to change your passwords to reflect your goals or the mind-set you're trying to cultivate. For example, if there's a word or phrase that sums up what you're working toward, something that makes you feel happy or uplifted, or even an income goal, work it in. It's a tiny drop in the bucket, but considering how many times per day we're asked to enter passwords, it can add up, big-time.

I spoke with holistic wealth coach and author of *Beau-*

tiful Money, Leanne Jacobs, about looking at the big picture of what you want—and why it's important to reframe your journey as a story about energy management.

Identify What You Want

Whoever came up with that business about "Don't say your wish out loud or it won't come true" was full of shit. Don't be afraid to get really, really clear about what you want to accomplish or what you want to see in your life. Similar to how we say, "Awareness is the first step," you have to declare what you want to manifest. Knowing where you want to go gives you a destination so you can ask yourself along the way, "Is this helping me get to where I want to be?"

Resist the Urge to Compartmentalize

We often look at themes like money, health, and relationships as separate, but Jacobs stresses, "It's about balance. Sometimes we get a little too hooked or attached to one particular dimension. Maybe we're overly attached to work or obsessed with nutrition to the point where we put ten labels on how we eat and who we are, which becomes unhealthy. Our goal is to remain open and flexible and kind and loving, and the more labels we put on ourselves, the more it makes our energy system brittle."

Everything is a part of a whole, she explains. When looking to make a change or manifest something we want, "It's about scanning our body and our life as well as scanning our fear and how our issues can affect health."

So if you're looking to manifest something in one area of your life, assess how other areas factor in. For example, when I was first trying to grow my private practice, I had to take an honest look at how some of my other work commitments were impacting my sleep habits, which in turn had an effect on how I came across at networking events, on calls with potential clients, and online in my blog and social media.

Make It About Energy

Jacobs believes we need to shift from being time managers to energy managers in order to get to our next level of prosperity, success, and health. "We need to graduate from hustling," she emphasizes. "Yes, we have to know how to manage time, but once you have that down, it's more about being mindful of where we hemorrhage energy and the poor choices that are keeping us unhealthy." You can be eating all the kale (or whatever stereotypically healthy food you can imagine) but if you're leaking energy and burning yourself out in other areas of your life, you're never going to get to that place of optimal wellness.

Expect That What You Want Is Coming

"We want to train and instruct the subconscious to command what we want"—not in a super controlling or fearful type of way, says Jacobs, but in a positive way that makes us feel excited and hopeful. When we're in that open-minded, optimistic state, we may have an easier time receiving or spotting next steps we might not notice if we were feeling down or burned out.

While I'm usually the first to roll my eyes at that Cinderella "someday-my-prince-will-come" thing, if you think about it, she so truly believed that this dude was on his way, you might say she manifested the situation that led her to make his acquaintance at the ball.

That doesn't mean you can be lazy or avoid putting in the work. For example, if Cinderella had told her fairy godmother to get lost or if she had refused to get in the pumpkin carriage and insisted her prince was supposed to literally come to her doorstep, the outcome of the story would have been quite different because she would have just sat at home waiting all night.

I mean, sure, we don't have real-life gourd wagons hauling us around, but being open to recognizing which things could lead us to our destination can be valuable. Maybe it's an invitation to an event that's intriguing but outside your comfort zone, maybe it's a chance meeting with someone new, maybe it's reading a line in a book that fell open on the floor that gives you a brilliant idea and propels you toward your goal.

Choose Your Tools
Any little tool that helps you expect that what you desire is on its way helps, explains Jacobs, so when you're feeling low-energy or slipping into a negative headspace, that tool can help us feel a little bit more hopeful so we stay in a positive, open mind-set.

There are so many tools you can use to help manifest things. You can try vision boards, affirmations, journaling, crystals, and plenty more where that came from. Choose what speaks to you.

Jacobs shares, "I like Kundalini mantras. I don't use them just for money, but I will pick one that may focus on abundance or on prosperity if that's how I feel that day. My phone is also always programmed with podcast episodes and e-books, so that when I'm on the go I can use those to program my subconscious toward prosperity and abundance."

She's also a fan of affirmations, often tweaking ones she likes so that the message rings true on a deeper level. If something you hear or read resonates with you, you can tweak it slightly so that it most accurately reflects what you want and how you want to feel. "When it's your own wording, your cells are going to believe it more than if you take someone else's because it sounds good." She also likes to use a tool like Canva, a graphic-design tool website, to make it look pretty.

And, like me, Jacobs is a fan of changing your passwords to reflect a specific goal, be it an income goal, a mind-set you want to cultivate, or something else that speaks to you.

Commit to New Wiring

"I think our caveman brain is wired to wait until there's a crisis to move," says Jacobs. "We're all good at being obsessively busy and chaotic. We don't need to work on that. I think we need to be more focused on the inner work of disciplining the five senses not to be unhealthily attached" to things that don't serve us.

"The brain is a muscle that has to be built," she adds. "It's new wiring we have to commit to, and it takes a lot of practice. It's a daily practice. One of my teachers said, 'The ego is really smart and very persistent.' We're going to make breaks and breakthroughs and feel really amazing, and then we'll have a day where our ego and our old habits take over and we feel like we're going backward, and we have to just learn to be at peace with the humanity of it all and not be so hard on ourselves."

Those challenging times, after all, can give us valuable insight into where we struggle (for example, how fear, stress, and anxiety can hijack our thought patterns and actions) so that we can learn helpful strategies to handle those situations.

Looking at how different facets of your life align with your values is another way to weed out what doesn't serve the big picture. "If we don't align with our values, we're doing a job we don't like, we're in a relationship that's toxic, or we're not taking care of ourselves, we'll get complacent, and it's easy to get stuck in that unhealthy space where we can't feel the fire" that keeps us self-motivated and confident. "I do believe there is a correlation between powerful self-motivation and self-esteem."

Make Rituals Part of Your Self-Care Routine

To be more magnetic, says Jacobs, "I truly believe that when we're taking care of our health and looking at the body, our energetic system is wider, denser," and helps attract what we desire.

"I believe that self-care rituals strengthen our energy system to a level that will draw the world in. If we're not taking care of ourselves, we likely won't draw what we desire to the same level or with the same speed that we would if we were feeling amazing."

Jacobs explains that, rather than getting lost going down the to-do-list and research rabbit holes, "If I'm looking to manifest something specific, I always start with my own energy system and ask myself, 'What do I need to shift inside to draw that into me?' I do feel that rituals in self-care are so much more powerful than we think."

An example she gives is that if someone is working on their financial health, "It may become a ritual practice for somebody to check their credit score each week" as just a part of their self-care upkeep, not unlike how we look at brushing our teeth or some similarly mundane activity.

One of her personal go-to rituals is, "When I'm feeling chaotic, I go to my drawer that holds my utility bills and I clean them out and pay them all off, and instantly I feel healthier. I consider that a health ritual more than a money ritual."

Keep It Simple

"It is sometimes hard to sustain if we do too many rituals," says Jacobs. As we talked about in the chapter on routine, you don't have to rise before dawn every morning to do a two-hour meditation or spend exorbitant amounts of money on treatments and gear.

Jacobs likes to point out that many of the best rituals are free—like drinking water or taking a bath. If yoga is your thing, you can find amazing low-cost and no-cost resources. Libraries are a great place for books.

Generally speaking, though, says Jacobs, "Anything that will lighten how dense we feel is a health practice."

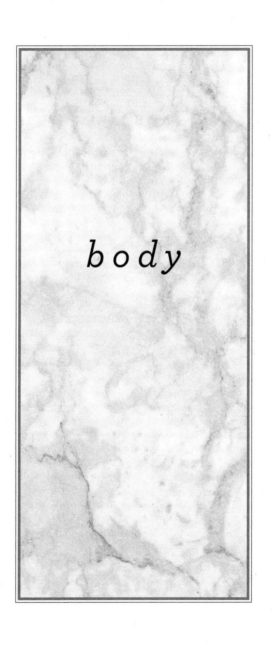

body

HANGER MANAGEMENT 101

Hunger + Anger = Hanger

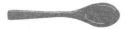

HAVE YOU EVER felt angry because you were hungry? Have you ever raged at a colleague, friend, or family member who politely asked you to please just eat something? If so, you've felt the sensation of hanger, and you know that it's no joke.

Low blood sugar is the main contributor to hanger, and, generally speaking, comes from waiting too long between meals, or from eating things that break down very quickly and don't fill us up. When we start feeling hangry, our energy, focus, productivity, and mood all take a hit.

How It Works

Carbohydrates—found in grains, fruit, starchy vegetables, and the like—raise our blood sugar. Protein, fat, and fiber counteract that effect by slowing digestion. When we eat a meal or snack that contains a combination of carbohydrates and protein and/or fat, we experience slower breakdown of the carbs, and, therefore, a more stable blood sugar level for a longer period of time after eating. This helps us feel more satisfied and energized and supports a more stable mood so we're less likely to want to bite someone's head off.

The lactose in milk products is also a form of carbohydrate, but how quickly it breaks down depends on whether it's in the context of a full-fat or low-fat dairy product. Cheese, for example, is essentially the protein and fat from milk, whereas the lactose in a glass of skim milk will hit the bloodstream more quickly and be broken down more rapidly.

When we eat carbs (especially refined or "simple" carbs like pastries, white bread, etc.) on an empty stomach, we get a sharp rise in glucose and insulin, followed shortly by a crash. That's why a donut or a plate of pancakes may leave you hungry again and ready for a nap an hour after eating. That's hardly going to help you get through a busy morning.

On the other hand, having a breakfast of, say, a slice of whole grain bread (whole grains, an example of a "complex" carbohydrate, digest more slowly than refined grains like white bread) with an egg (which provides protein and fat) and half an avocado (a great source of both fat and fiber) will help us feel satisfied and alert for several hours. This helps us focus and have a more productive day. It also makes us less likely to want to smack a colleague for talking too loudly or having an annoying sneeze. It helps us have smoother interactions with others we encounter throughout our day.

Friends and Frenemies

When it comes to nourishment and stable blood sugar, it's important to know the difference between "friends"—typically unprocessed foods—which do you favors by providing lots of nutrients, and "frenemies"—foods that might seem fun and nice, but which ultimately make you feel like crap.

While your diet doesn't have to consist 100 percent of friends, they should make up the majority of your diet. A 90:10 or 80:20 ratio of nourishing, healthy foods to treats can be a sustainable balance to strive for.

Foods That Do You Favors:

- Fruits
- Vegetables
- Nuts and nut butters: almonds, hazelnuts, pistachios, walnuts, peanuts (technically legumes but have a similar nutritional profile) etc.
- Seeds and seed butters: pumpkin, sunflower, sesame, chia, flax, hemp, etc.
- Avocados
- Eggs
- Fish
- Lean meats: chicken, turkey, lean beef, and pork
- Beans, peas, lentils
- Whole grains

- Dairy: yogurt, cheese, and milk*
- Unrefined oils: olive, avocado, and sesame oil

Frenemy Foods:

- Added sugar (this can include its many forms, such as cane sugar, fructose, sucrose, dextrose, etc.)
- Artificial sweeteners (a few common ones include aspartame and sucralose)
- Refined grains (pastries, white bread, white pasta, etc.)
- Processed snacks like chips and cookies with lots of preservatives and other additives
- Trans fats (partially hydrogenated oils)
- Foods with artificial coloring or dyes

You'll notice I left some things off the "frenemy" list (butter, bacon, honey, lamb, maple syrup, to name a few), and that's because these are things on the "in moderation" list, meaning that regularly consuming them as part of your daily diet may not be healthy, but it doesn't mean you can't *ever* eat those things—they're just better off as an occasional treat. They may even offer some nutritional benefits—but the amount and frequency matters. Lamb, for example, is a great

---

* People who are lactose intolerant don't tolerate dairy well and may wish to avoid it. It's also okay if you follow a vegan or dairy-free diet—just be mindful to cover your nutritional bases to account for that. There are plenty of alternate ways to get the nutrients found in milk from other sources. For example, you can get calcium from tofu and certain leafy green vegetables like broccoli and bok choy, or from a fortified nondairy product.

source of protein and iron, but a high intake of red meat has been linked to colorectal cancers.

Think of the frenemies as foods that really aren't offering any nutritional benefits and that might make you feel uncomfortable afterward. I want to be cautious about saying you should never eat them—more so, it's just important to know what you're dealing with. I don't consider any particular food "evil" or something to put permanently off-limits if it's something you truly love. You just need to be mindful about making it part of an experience you'll actually savor and can move on from, rather than going down a food-guilt spiral.

The key is that including more of the foods that do you favors in the context of your diet will help you feel healthy and stable, but still leaves room for other things you enjoy simply for pleasure. For example, maybe you're roasting nutrient-rich brussels sprouts to eat with your baked salmon, but then you add a crumbled strip of bacon to the batch for extra flavor.

As far as liquids go, water is your best bet for hydration, but if you want something a little different, seltzer is a great alternative. If you just can't get into the unflavored stuff, squeeze in some citrus or add a splash of juice.

Coffee and tea are beverages that have been shown to have some potential health benefits but may not be appropriate for everyone. You're the expert on you, so be honest with yourself about how caffeine impacts you.

Alcohol is another beverage that's been noted for some

positive effects, but again, limit yourself to an amount that's appropriate for you. Current recommendations are for men to stick to two or fewer alcoholic drinks per day, and for women to consume one or fewer. If you're not sure what one drink looks like, that's either 12 ounces of beer, 5 ounces of wine, or 1 ounce of spirits.[18]

Portions Count

The ratio of carbs to protein to fat also plays a role in how quickly a meal breaks down. If you go online looking for information on the exact ratio to eat to be healthy, you'll get an overwhelming amount of opinions, some of which have more grounding in science than others. Pay attention to which foods and combinations of foods make you feel energized and satisfied and which ones make you feel more prone to hanger.

Just because some random person on social media who lost a lot of weight says she feels like a magical unicorn eating a certain way, it doesn't mean that what worked for her will get your body to function at its peak. We'll talk more about this later, but as a general guideline, though, aim to fill half of your lunch and dinner plate with non-starchy vegetables, a quarter with protein, and a quarter with carbohydrates.

WANT TO TRUST YOUR GUT? TAKE CARE OF IT.

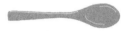

WE SO OFTEN hear and use the phrases "trust your gut" or "gut feeling," but have you ever really thought about what they truly mean? And then of course there's the term "nervous stomach." Think about it—when you've been under a lot of stress or something scares you, have you found yourself rushing to the bathroom or noticed that you had completely lost your appetite?

As it turns out, the gastrointestinal system and the brain communicate with each other via the gut-brain connection.[19]

I spoke with Dr. Taz Bhatia, a board-certified doctor in integrative medicine and author of *Super Woman Rx*, about gut health and how it's truly the foundation of our overall mental, emotional, and physical health.

What Is the Gut-Brain Connection, Anyway?

Dr. Taz explains, "The digestive system is the foundation of health, something eastern systems of medicine like Chinese medicine and Ayurveda harped on thousands of years ago. Today, in research we are seeing how digestive health—

based on the gut microbiome; the balance of gut bacteria, digestion, and absorption of fat; and the integrity of the gut lining—impact inflammation, the gut-brain connection, and the ability to detoxify."

The gut is like a second brain that lines your gastrointestinal tract, all the way from the esophagus to the rectum. It has a name, too—the *enteric nervous system* (ENS)—and is comprised of two thin layers. It's estimated to have anywhere between over 200 and 600 million nerve cells.[20]

In short, what goes on in your gastrointestinal (GI) system can impact your brain function and play a role in your cognitive function and mental health—and vice versa. The health of the gut microbiome (the communities of bacteria that live in the gut) directly impacts how effectively our body absorbs and utilizes the nutrients in the food we eat, which in turn can impact the brain's physiological, behavioral, and cognitive functions, because some of the major mood-regulating neurotransmitters like serotonin are produced in the gut.

A lot of our immune system function also takes place in the gut, as those gut bacteria interact with invading pathogens.[21]

Nurturing the health of your gut is one of the best ways to take care of your brain and support stable mental health and sharp cognitive function.

While anxiety and stress can cause GI disturbances and contribute to conditions like irritable bowel syndrome (IBS), when GI problems interrupt our daily activities, they can become the cause of our stress and anxiety. And stress further suppresses your immune system, making it hard for your body to fight off subsequent infections.[22]

Think about how this connection plays out for you. For example, have you ever noticed that after you get sick and have to miss a lot of work time, catching up adds a lot of new stress and you find yourself struggling to feel well again?

"I think many people medicate individual symptoms like constipation or diarrhea, without trying to find the root cause and treat the whole picture or balance needed in the digestive tract," says Dr. Taz. Watch for telltale signs that your gut health might be out of alignment, such as "irregularity in bowel habits including constipation, diarrhea, or change in digestive symptoms like bloating, reflux, or pain." These could all signify that you need to pay more attention to what's going on in your gut and take steps to address the issue.

What to Feed Your Gut

If you want to trust your gut, you should take care of it. Nurturing our gut health with the right foods can go a long way in supporting our overall wellness.

Probiotics

Probiotics are beneficial gut bacteria. There are many different varieties that perform different functions. They support regular digestion, impact nutrient utilization, and are part of immune system function. To keep your gut healthy, it's important to get your probiotics from a variety of sources, so mix up food sources. We'll talk about supplements below. Here are some of the sources I recommend most to my clients:

- **Yogurt** is one of the most approachable probiotic-rich foods. You can eat it for breakfast or a snack or use it in dressings and marinades. To get the most bang for your buck without the negative effect of sugar, artificial flavors, preservatives, or other additives, try to avoid the sweetened varieties and instead add your own cinnamon, honey, maple syrup, or fruit. If you don't eat dairy, there are a lot of cultured nondairy options on the market, but check the label to see what's in there.
- **Kefir** is another fermented dairy product that has a slightly tangier flavor and a thinner consistency than yogurt. Because it's very low in lactose (most varieties are about 99 percent lactose-free), people who are sensitive to other dairy products may find they tolerate kefir without a problem. You can enjoy it on its own or add it to smoothies, a bowl of cereal, or use it to make overnight oats—more on that one later.
- **Kimchi** is a traditional Korean food that's made by fermenting vegetables with lactic acid bacteria. It's a delicious garnish for salads and stir-fry dishes. You can also eat it plain.
- **Sauerkraut** is made of fermented cabbage and is

part of many traditional Central European dishes. To ensure that you're getting live bacteria, choose a product that's sold in the refrigerated section, and don't panic if you hear it hissing and fizzing when you open the jar—that's a totally normal part of the fermentation process, which actually continues even after packaging. Enjoy sauerkraut in a sandwich, tossed into salad, or as a topping for eggs or grain bowls.

- **Miso** is a fermented soybean paste with a smooth texture and salty flavor that's used frequently in Asian cooking. The most common varieties of miso you'll see in stores are typically white, yellow, and red. You can use miso paste to make dressings, sauces, marinades, and soup bases. Just note that miso is not gluten-free, as the soybeans are typically fermented with barley and sometimes other grains. Avoid this one if you're gluten-sensitive or trying to avoid gluten.
- **Kombucha** is a fermented tea beverage with a tangy flavor and fizzy texture. Bear in mind that many traditional and commercial recipes call for sugar, so scope out the label to see how much. If it's more than 10 grams per bottle, enjoy it over the course of a couple days instead of in one sitting. Also important to note: Kombucha does contain a tiny amount of alcohol (around 0.5 percent) and caffeine, so take that into account if you're sensitive.

Prebiotics

Prebiotics are foods—usually high in fiber—that serve as food for probiotic bacteria, so to speak.[23] Having adequate sources of prebiotics in your diet helps promote an increase in probiotic bacteria.

A few good sources of prebiotics include:

- Apples
- Artichokes
- Asparagus
- Bananas
- Barley
- Chicory root
- Dark chocolate
- Garlic
- Jerusalem artichokes
- Leeks
- Oats
- Onions
- Wheat bran

Other Foods That Support Gut Health

In general, consuming enough fiber can also support digestive health by promoting regular bowel movements. Current recommendations are 25-35 grams per day for most healthy adults. Some good sources of dietary fiber include whole grains, beans, legumes, vegetables, fruits, nuts, and seeds. There are two types of fiber: soluble and insoluble. Soluble fiber, when combined with water, forms a gel of sorts, which takes up space in the stomach and slows digestion. Some good sources include beans, apples, pears, oats, oat bran, barley, flax, sweet potatoes, and avocados. Insoluble fiber helps form stool bulk and helps food move through the GI tract. A few foods you can find it in include vegetables, nuts, seeds, and whole grains.

Researchers have also looked at bone broth and its potential to support gut health. It's easy to digest and provides a variety of vitamins, minerals, and important amino acids that support the healthy repair of tissue lining the GI tract. Specifically, the gelatin in bone broth has also been associated with an improvement in the integrity of the gut—meaning that it helps ensure that the lining of the intestinal tract is healthy and intact, and that it provides a secure barrier to keep bacteria in the GI tract from seeping out into the bloodstream.[24] When that barrier is functioning properly, it allows water and nutrients to pass through but prevents harmful substances from doing so.

Additionally, amino acids proline,[25] glycine,[26] and glutamine,[27] which are present in bone broth, have been associated with improved gut health. Bone broth also contains collagen,[28] which has been noted for its benefit to the intestinal lining.

While I wouldn't suggest that you replace all of your water intake with bone broth, it can be part of a gut-healthy diet. If drinking a mug of hot, savory liquid feels weird to you, try using it as a base for homemade soups instead.

In addition to probiotic-rich foods and bone broth, Dr. Taz also recommends consuming adequate healthy fats. MCT oil is one of her go-to sources, but you can also use other healthy fats like avocados and olive oil. Among the many known health benefits, research in animals has shown that both avocado[29] and olive oils[30] may improve gut microbiota (the bacteria that live in the gut).

How to Use Supplements

I'm not a supplement-pusher, but I make a few exceptions, and probiotics are on my short list. Making probiotic supplements part of your wellness routine is one of the easiest ways to support gut health, especially if you're not consistent with your intake of probiotic-rich foods. Because the different types of probiotic bacteria have different functions in the body, look for a supplement with a variety of bacteria as opposed to just one strain to ensure you cover more bases. A few must-have bacteria strains, Dr. Taz says, are lactobacillus, bifido bacteria, and saccharomyces boulardii.

There is a lot of confusion about the optimal number of bacteria to aim for. You'll commonly see amounts from 1 to 10 billion CFUs (Colony Forming Units) on supplement bottles. Reading labels can make your head spin. Is more necessarily better? You'll get different answers depending on whom you ask and which brands you're considering. A lot also depends on what you're trying to achieve by taking that supplement—are you trying to heal an acute issue or is your goal to support a baseline healthy gut microbiome? What I usually tell my clients is to purchase a multi-strain product with a CFU count between 4 and 10 billion and to increase the dose if they need more. However, for a specific health condition, consulting with a gastrointestinal specialist can be valuable.

While many shelf-stable varieties are now available, some may need to be refrigerated after opening. Ask your pharmacist if you're not sure. And while serious side effects are very rare, Dr. Taz says to pay attention to any side effects like bloating or diarrhea, and to ask your doctor or pharmacist about any potential interference with prescribed medications.

Some supplements may provide a combination of probiotics and prebiotics, so check out your available options. What works for one person may not be the right fit for someone else. If you know you don't get a lot of prebiotics from food sources, that's probably the place to start.

Bottom Line

The health of your gastrointestinal system has a definite impact on your physiological, behavioral, and emotional health. Consuming a variety of prebiotics and probiotic-rich foods can help support gut health. Supplements are also available if you need help being consistent.

EAT TO
BEAT STRESS

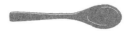

STRESS CAN HAVE a huge impact on our eating behavior. For some people, stress and/or anxiety causes a loss of appetite. But many overeat and struggle to make progress with their dietary goals because they find themselves turning to food when they feel like their nervous system is short-circuiting.

If you're quick to make stress-eating a story about lacking willpower or just being bad at taking care of yourself, you might want to rethink that. Stress-related appetite changes are actually a physiological response.[31] In the short term, the brain tells the kidneys to release epinephrine (aka adrenaline), triggering a fight-or-flight response that temporarily shuts down our perception of hunger. If you've ever had to deal with an emergency situation and didn't realize you hadn't eaten until hours later, yet you can't seem to make it through an hour on your average workday without grazing, that's likely the mechanism that was at work.

On the flip side, when that stress continues (for example,

when you're dealing with the slow-burning soul-suck of a toxic work environment or a drawn-out situation in your personal or professional life that gnaws at you 24/7), your adrenal glands release the stress hormone cortisol, which can both increase your appetite and amp up your desire to eat. On a primal level, your brain is trying to increase your motivation to survive in the face of a perceived threat, but it doesn't realize you're just sitting at a desk. Though cortisol levels are supposed to go back down once the stressful episode concludes, when the stress continues, cortisol levels can stay elevated, leading to inflammation.

Human and animal studies have also looked at stress-induced changes in preference for food, and it turns out that we tend to reach for highly palatable comfort foods, especially those high in fat and sugar. Some researchers believe that increased levels of cortisol, insulin, and/or the hunger hormone ghrelin are the culprits.

While food is obviously a big piece of this picture, it's also worth noting that during stressful periods, people tend to exercise less and drink more alcohol—two things that can contribute to weight gain, especially when combined with an increase of calories. Sleep disturbances are another common issue with stress, and when we're short on shut-eye, changes in our leptin and ghrelin levels make us more aware of our hunger and less in tune with feelings of fullness and satisfaction. Lose-lose situation.

The good news is that even if we can't directly control the things that stress us out, what we eat can improve our stress response so we can feel more grounded and better able to handle the craziness coming at us.

Make It About Blood Sugar

When it comes to keeping our shit together during times of stress, blood sugar management is key. Meals and snacks that provide a combination of protein, fat, and complex carbohydrates break down slowly so we don't get that crash-and-burn feeling that comes from eating simple carbs like chips, pastries, and candy—or that meltdown-y feeling that comes from skipping meals or forgetting to eat until we've reached the point of no return.

To share a personal example, when I was in New York working at the hospital during Hurricane Sandy in 2012, it was one of the most stressful experiences I had ever faced. I felt out of touch with my hunger until I'd completely hit a wall and turned into a raging, shaky beast.

There was one morning when I had a very short break. I could either have had a snack or made a phone call to tell my mom I was okay, like I'd promised I would. I went with the snack, and I was so hangry, the rubbery hard-boiled egg from the cafeteria's emergency stash was basically the best thing I had ever eaten. I actually hadn't known until that moment that I even liked hard-boiled eggs.

Sanity restored, I was able to dive back into the day, and I realized that—duh—I could text my mom to say all was chaotic but safe. That week was actually a lightbulb moment for me in terms of learning about the importance of stabilizing blood sugar in order to keep it together at work and in stressful situations.

Stress-Busting Superfoods

Speaking of eggs, they're just one of several foods that have specific compounds that can help support a healthy stress response. Here are the stress-busting foods I most often recommend to clients:

- **Eggs** are rich in choline,[32] a nutrient that's essential to brain function. The combination of protein and fat is also very grounding. Make it a balanced meal by enjoying eggs with a complex carbohydrate source like roasted sweet potatoes or whole grain toast.
- **Sweet potatoes** are a good source of complex carbs, which are important for efficient production of the mood-regulating neurotransmitter serotonin, as they promote insulin release, which boosts absorption of the amino acid tryptophan, a precursor to serotonin. You can chop them up and roast a big batch to enjoy through the week, or for a shortcut version, prick one a few times with a fork and microwave until soft on the inside. Enjoy with a sprinkle of goat cheese or a smear of nut butter or tahini for a delicious twist on a baked potato.
- **Dark, leafy greens** are a good source of folate,[33] a B-vitamin that helps support efficient production of the feel-good brain chemical dopamine. Add spinach

to a smoothie, enjoy a big arugula salad, sneak some greens onto a sandwich, or sauté up some chard or kale to enjoy with your favorite protein. You can also easily add greens to soups, stews, and more.

- **Avocados** are a good source of heart-healthy mono-unsaturated fat as well as fiber, both of which help slow digestion so you can feel satisfied longer and avoid any hanger management issues. Avocado toast with a side salad is a delicious example of a simple, grounding meal. Add an egg on top for extra satisfying protein and fat plus brain-boosting choline.

- **Plain yogurt** provides beneficial probiotic bacteria to support a healthy gut-brain connection. It's also a good source of protein to keep you satisfied. Skipping the flavored stuff saves you the blood sugar roller coaster that often comes with sugary versions. It also provides calcium,[34] a mineral that's important for muscle and nerve function and efficient cell signaling—important for regulation of those neurotransmitters. Enjoy it as the base for a yogurt bowl or add it to a smoothie.

- **Berries** are one of my go-to fruits because there's so much to love. They're packed with fiber as well as vitamin C. The antioxidants in berries have also been associated with anti-inflammatory and other benefits that help protect the body from the damage caused by chronic stress.[35] I especially love frozen berries because you can enjoy the nutritional benefits year-round, as they're frozen at peak freshness and retain all their nutritious goodness. You can thaw them in the fridge or microwave, or just eat them still frozen. I personally think that frozen berries are delicious with Greek yogurt.

- **Salmon** and other fatty fish like tuna, mackerel, and sardines, are rich in omega-3 fatty acids, which are helpful for taming the impact of the stress hormone cortisol and promoting improved mood and cognitive function.[36] Animal proteins, fish included, are all good sources of tryptophan as well.

- **Oats** are a plant-based source of tryptophan, and an affordable, versatile whole grain option to keep handy. A bowl of oats with nut butter and berries makes a delicious, easy breakfast, but you can also go savory by using spices like garlic, turmeric, ginger, and paprika and top your bowl with veggies and an egg and some healthy fat, such as tahini or avocado slices. Use oats as a substitute for breadcrumbs in meatballs and meatloaf, or throw them into a smoothie. You can also use them to make your own healthy granola or baked goods.

- **Olive oil** Even if I wasn't half Italian and Greek, I'd be enthusiastic about this one. Aside from being delicious, it's one of the most studied anti-inflammatory foods and is an excellent source of heart-healthy monounsaturated fat that's been shown to help reduce the effects of oxidative stress.[37] Make extra virgin olive oil your go-to for salad dressings, marinades, and cooking.

- **Turmeric** is an herb that's been used medicinally for thousands of years to treat a wide range of ailments. Curcumin, the active compound in turmeric, has been touted for its anti-inflammatory, antioxidant properties. It's also been shown to have a lot of potential to benefit mental health.[38] You can add this one to soups, stews, curries, sauces, marinades, or salad dressings. Or use it to make a tea with ginger and black pepper.

- **Dark chocolate** has been widely studied for the anti-inflammatory and antioxidant properties of the powerful compounds it contains called flavonoids. Research has suggested that chocolate (at least 85 percent cacao, specifically) may be helpful for lowering cortisol levels and reducing perceived stress.[39] Just pay attention to portions. About an ounce per day is all you need—and that's within the context of your daily calorie intake.

Bottom Line

What you eat can improve your stress response. Make sure you're consuming balanced meals and snacks. Incorporating foods with stress-fighting properties as a regular part of your diet can further support your stress management.

DON'T FEAR FAT

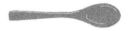

AS AN ELDER millennial, I lived a good portion of my formative years without the Internet, and can still remember when avocados and olive oil were looked at as "fattening" and SnackWell's cookies were considered health food. My grandmother used to buy fat-free cheese, and I'm a little afraid to think about what was even in that stuff. Amazing how things have changed!

While I learned in nutrition school about the importance of dietary fat, I gained a strong appreciation for its power the winter I turned thirty-two and felt like my life was falling apart. My dad was very ill at the time, and I was so worn out from rushing back and forth between New York, New Jersey, and whatever hospital or doctor's office he happened to be in on whatever day, my immune system took a major hit. My cortisol levels were a little elevated, thanks to the mental and emotional stress, not to mention the toll all that stress took on my sleep.

It was also during this time that I found myself on four rounds of antibiotics to heal an infection in my left thumbnail, which ended up needing to be removed. The gut-brain connection we talked about a few chapters ago? Um, yeah—because antibiotics kill all the good bacteria with the bad, I was in rough shape. I had no energy and felt like I just couldn't think straight, much less communicate clearly.

I was trying so hard to keep it together for my family, but when an allergic reaction to one of those antibiotics led to me having to get an emergency Benadryl shot and lie on the couch thinking about my own mortality for an entire day, I had to get real about the fact that something wasn't working. It was a slow burn of a near-death experience, but still, very much a wake-up call.

As I got my health back on track, it seemed like all I wanted to eat was hard-boiled eggs and arugula salad with avocado, wild sardines packed in olive oil, and radishes cooked in butter. For snacks, I was all about whole milk Greek yogurt with sunflower seed butter and frozen berries. Something was up—and no, I wasn't pregnant. I started exploring these cravings more and realized that a lot of these foods were rich in important fatty acids my brain and body were crying out for.

Here's what I mean.

Why Fat Is Important

The thing is, we actually need fat in our diet. Fat provides energy, protects our organs, and plays a vital role in body functions such as temperature regulation, hormone production, and cell growth. Fat is also part of the structure of cells, including brain cells. Having adequate fat in the diet has also been linked to better cognitive function. Certain fats like omega-3 fatty acids have been shown to counter the inflammatory effect of stress in the body.[40]

Having fat in our diet is also really important for feeling satisfied, as we talked about in the Hanger Management chapter. Even a little can go a long way toward giving a meal or snack staying power that will keep us full and energized for a long time.

One gram of fat, regardless of the type, contains 9 calories. But not all fats are equal. There are actually several different types of fat, each of which has a different structure and behaves somewhat differently in the body.[41] They are:

- Saturated Fat
- Trans Fat
- Monounsaturated Fat
- Polyunsaturated Fat

Saturated and trans fats are what you'll often see called "bad" fats, and they're generally solid at room temperature. They have been shown to raise LDL cholesterol (the "bad" cholesterol).

Saturated fat is generally found in foods like fatty beef, lamb, poultry with skin, egg yolks, and dairy, as well as in coconut oil. It used to be thought that we should avoid these foods as much as possible, but recent research has suggested that as long as you're consuming them in amounts to suit your goals, they can be a part of a healthy diet.

There's a lot of conflicting information about coconut oil. While it's a saturated fat, the primary fatty acid found in coconut oil, lauric acid, is a medium-chain fatty acid that has 12 carbon atoms. All triglyceride molecules are composed of three fatty acid molecules and a glycerol molecule. Medium-chain triglycerides, which are made from fatty acids with 6-12 carbon atoms, are processed by the body differently from other fats, and may produce a variety of health benefits, from weight loss to improved brain function, according to some research. That said, there are several other types of fatty acids in coconut oil.[42]

While I do think that coconut oil can be a part of a healthy diet, as with anything, too much of a good thing can be a bad thing. Context and portions still count with this one. I generally encourage consuming coconut oil in the context of your saturated fat intake for the day. More on that below.

I usually tell my clients to avoid trans fats, though, as this one both raises LDL and lowers HDL ("good") cholesterol. Trans fats are found in many commercial baked goods as well as in fried foods, margarine, and some dressings, sauces, and the like. Check labels to make sure. A red flag is seeing "partially hydrogenated" oil on the ingredients label. This means that hydrogen atoms have been added to the fatty acids to make them solid at room temperature and, therefore, more shelf-stable.

Monounsaturated and polyunsaturated fats are often referred to as the "good" fats, and are generally liquid at room temperature. They have been shown to help lower LDL ("bad") cholesterol and increase HDL ("good") cholesterol. Good food sources of monounsaturated fats include olive oil, canola oil, safflower oil, avocados, and many nuts and seeds.

Sources of polyunsaturated fat include sunflower oil, soybean oil, and corn oil.

If you're wondering where omega-3s fit in, here you go. Omega-3 fatty acids are a type of polyunsaturated fat.[43] There are three types, including:

- *eicosapentaenoic acid (EPA)*, a 20-carbon fatty acid that's involved in the production of chemicals called eicosanoids, which help reduce inflammation in the body.[44] EPA has also been associated with decreased symptoms of depression.[45] Food sources include fatty fish like salmon, tuna, sardines, and mackerel.
- *docosahexaenoic acid (DHA)*, a 22-carbon fatty acid that's essential for normal fetal brain development[46] and proper brain function in adults and children.[47] You'll find it in a lot of the same fish as EPA.
- *alpha-linolenic acid (ALA)*, an 18-carbon, plant-based omega-3 fatty acid that's a precursor to EPA and DHA. This means that ALA we consume can be converted into EPA and DHA in the body. However, the process isn't very efficient, so someone on a plant-based diet would need to consume a larger amount or use a supplement to get an amount close to what they would get if they were consuming food sources of EPA

and DHA. Because it's the only one of the three that our body can't make on its own, ALA is considered an essential fatty acid. Food sources of ALA include flaxseed and flaxseed oil, chia seeds, and walnuts.

How Much Fat Do You Need?

The exact amount of dietary fat required can vary from person to person. For example, a doctor may recommend a low-fat diet for certain gastrointestinal conditions like pancreatitis, or a very high-fat diet for someone with a neurological condition like drug-resistant epilepsy. Have you heard of the keto diet? It was started in the 1920s to treat epilepsy long before it was a weight loss fad. For someone with a heart condition or who has an elevated risk of heart disease, special attention may be paid to the specific sources of dietary fat, like limiting saturated fat while promoting mono- and polyunsaturated fats.

The 2015-2020 *Dietary Guidelines for Americans* recommends consuming 20-35 percent of your total calories from fat, with no more than 10 percent of your daily calories coming from saturated fat. For someone on a 2,000-calorie diet, that's about 200 calories, or just over 22 grams of saturated fat per day.[48] The American Heart Association is slightly more conservative, recommending that your saturated fat intake account for just 5 to 6 percent of your calories—11 to 13 grams for someone on a 2,000-calorie diet.[49]

While there are no set requirements for omega-3 fatty acids, it's generally recommended that healthy adults consume about 1.1-1.6 grams per day, though this is actually the recommendation for ALA, since that's the only omega-3 fatty acid that's essential. If you're regularly consuming fish you'll hit that target a lot more quickly. Eating fish two to three times per week can help you cover all of your omega-3 bases.[50]

Becoming aware of how much fat keeps you feeling satisfied and energized can help you find your sweet spot.

In general, spreading fat throughout your day in appropriate serving sizes can help you enjoy the benefits without overdoing it. Here are some examples.

How to Fit Healthy Fats Into Your Everyday Diet

At Breakfast

- Spread a quarter to a half of an avocado on whole grain toast and top with a fried or poached egg
- Enjoy a vegetable omelet made with whole eggs or top a bowl of veggies with eggs
- Add nut butter or nuts to a bowl of oatmeal
- Swap nut butter or tahini for butter on toast

At Lunch

- Add avocado to a salad
- Skip bottled low-fat salad dressing and make a simple vinaigrette with up to a tablespoon of extra virgin olive oil

- Enjoy a peanut butter and jelly sandwich on whole grain bread for a quick and easy lunch

At Dinner

- Make a walnut-based pesto to toss with pasta
- Enjoy baked salmon with your favorite vegetables and whole grain or starchy vegetable
- Roast veggies in olive, avocado, or sesame oil

At Snacks

- Hit up oyster happy hour with your friends for an omega-3 fix
- Enjoy nuts, seeds, or a nut-based bar as a portable snack
- Enjoy half an avocado with a dash of sea salt and a sprinkle of hemp seeds right from the skin, with the spoon.

Bottom Line

Don't fear fat. As part of a balanced diet, it's a crucial part of efficient brain function and energy management. Space out your intake through your day and include a variety of sources. If you need some guidance as to whether you need to limit saturated fat, consult with a registered dietitian.

EASY WAYS TO UP YOUR PROTEIN INTAKE

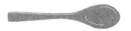

AS WE TOUCHED on in the chapter on Hanger Management, protein is an important nutrient for giving your meals and snacks staying power and ensuring that you keep your energy and mood on an even keel through the day.

On a cellular level, protein provides the amino acids that serve as building blocks for tissue growth and repair and support efficient function and regulation of numerous processes throughout the body.[51]

Of the 20 amino acids we get from plant and animal proteins, nine are considered essential, which means that our body can't synthesize them on its own and we need to get them from the foods that we eat (or from supplements). The essential amino acids include histidine, isoleucine, leucine, lysine, methionine, phenylalanine, threonine, tryptophan, and valine.

How Much Protein Do I Need?
Protein recommendations are based on about how much we need to consume to cover our needs for these essential

amino acids. Current protein recommendations for most healthy adults are 0.8-1.0 grams of protein per kilogram of body weight. One kilogram is equivalent to 2.2 pounds, so a 150-pound person (68.2 kilograms) needs about 55 to 68 grams of protein per day, according to those recommendations.[52]

There are different factors that can impact our needs, though. For example, if you're pregnant or nursing, are healing from an injury or surgery, or have a medical condition that increases your protein needs, you should have more. Athletes and very active individuals also generally require more protein to help support efficient muscle recovery and growth.

On the flip side, certain health conditions that impact the way your body metabolizes protein, such as kidney disease, may mean that you need to limit protein to a range closer to 0.6-0.8 grams per kilogram, depending on the severity. Ask your doctor or consult a registered dietitian if you need guidance on this one.

Just as a heads-up, someone on a vegetarian diet would likely need to consume closer to the higher end of that 0.8-1.0 grams per kilogram range, as it may take more work to cover their amino acid needs, since most plant protein sources provide some but not all of the amino acids we need to consume.

Some foods are considered "complete" proteins in that they have all nine essential amino acids. These tend to be animal sources of protein, with a few exceptions, including soy, quinoa, and buckwheat. However, combining different plant foods can help you cover your bases. For example, peanut butter and whole grain bread both provide some of the essential amino acids, and when you eat them together, you get all of the different ones you need. Same goes for rice and beans.

If the number of grams of protein you need sounds intimidating, break it down by meals and snacks to make that goal more attainable. For example, if someone needs 60 grams of protein per day, they could break that down into 20 grams per meal or 15 grams per meal with the remaining 15 grams coming from snacks.

What Foods Provide Protein?

A lot of people think that meat is the only protein source, but there are lots of great plant-based options as well.

Animal Sources of Protein:

- Meat
- Poultry
- Fish
- Eggs
- Milk and dairy products

Plant Sources of Protein:

- Beans
- Peas
- Lentils
- Nuts and nut butters
- Seeds and seed butters
- Soy products such as tofu, tempeh, and soy milk
- Nutritional yeast

Easy Ways to Add Protein to Your Day

Here are a few ideas to get you started.

At Breakfast:

- Top your toast with nut butter, ricotta, cottage cheese, or an egg instead of butter
- Enjoy a vegetable omelet
- Use milk or a protein-rich nondairy milk like pea or soy milk in hot or cold cereal
- Add a spoonful of nut or seed butter on top of a bowl of oatmeal
- Cook eggs or egg whites into oatmeal or stir in a scoop of protein powder at the end of cooking
- Use plain Greek yogurt as the base for a bowl with fruit and nuts or a green smoothie
- Add a serving of nuts to a bowl of cold cereal

At Lunch:

- Add cooked chicken, fish, tofu, eggs, or beans to a salad
- Enjoy a broth-based vegetable soup with beans in it
- Have cooked chicken, turkey, tofu, or hard-boiled egg on a sandwich

At Dinner:

- Add cooked fish, chicken, or sausage to a pasta dish
- Use bean- or lentil-based pasta for a meat-free, gluten-free alternative that's high in filling fiber as well as protein
- Enjoy your favorite cooked animal or plant protein with a side of cooked veggies and a starch like brown rice, quinoa, or sweet potato
- Add cooked ground turkey, leftover chicken, beans, or an egg to a vegetarian soup. You can also stir in unflavored protein powder
- Puréed or mashed white beans make a delicious high-protein, high-fiber side dish to a plate of green veggies

At Snacks:

- Enjoy a string cheese, cheese stick, or 1-oz serving of your favorite cheese with fruit or whole grain crackers

THE LITTLE BOOK OF GAME CHANGERS

- Enjoy a serving of plain Greek yogurt, ricotta, or cottage cheese with berries
- Have a minimally processed nut- or seed-based bar
- Have a stick of jerky as an easy snack
- Two hard-boiled eggs are a convenient snack that provides about 150 calories and about 12 grams of protein
- Enjoy a latte or cappuccino made with cow's milk or a protein-rich nondairy alternative—just keep in mind that many sugary versions will tack on a lot of extra calories, as will sweetened nondairy milks. Your best bet is a small size of an unsweetened beverage and to skip add-ons like syrups and whipped cream toppings.

Do You Need Protein Powder?

I get a lot of questions from clients about protein powder. Do you need it? Is it worth the money? How should you use it?

I know this is never the sexy, quick-fix answer anyone wants, but it really does depend on your unique situation. I generally encourage turning to food first to get the protein you need. However, if you have a chronic or acute medical condition that either increases your protein needs or impairs your ability to consume enough, protein powder might be helpful. For example, pregnancy and recovery from a surgical procedure are a few times you may need some help getting over the hump. If you've just had dental work or are dealing with a sore throat and need to stick to soft textures for a few days, protein powder can make smoothies, soups, and nice cream bowls (a nondairy alternative to ice cream, usually made with frozen banana in a blender or food processor) more substantial.

On a more serious note, in the case of someone with a condition like ALS that both impacts their ability to chew and swallow while also increasing their protein and calorie needs, protein powder can make a huge difference in helping them get what they need.

If you're someone who's on the go or travels a lot or who has an unpredictable schedule, protein powder can be a handy backup option to tide you over until you can have a regular meal. When I worked clinical, for example, plain instant oatmeal with protein powder made for an easy breakfast or even a snack. Today, I often carry a stick of collagen powder (a protein powder I like, in part because it just melts right in without adding a gritty texture or weird aftertaste) in my purse when I know I'll be out all day or traveling so that I can easily stir it into my coffee if I need a little boost to keep me going.

Protein powder can also be fun to play around with in homemade energy bars, fudge, and baked goods if you're looking for some more satisfying options and want to save money and avoid highly processed items in stores.

Just bear in mind that not all protein powders are created equal, so choose something that best suits your needs and preferences. Whey protein is a palatable option that's easy to find at many budget levels, but look for organic or grass-fed—it's worth the money. It's milk-based, so if you're lactose intolerant or have other issues with dairy products, this might not be the best option for you. Egg white protein is a great nondairy alternative that will lend a soft, fluffy texture to whatever you add it to. On the plant-based side, pea protein is super versatile and has a mild taste and texture. There are also a lot of great plant protein blends on the market. The main one I would encourage avoiding, though, is soy protein isolate, as it's more processed and no longer has the good parts of the soy plant—just the "filler" protein that allows companies that use it to be, like, "OMG, look how much protein we could fit in here!"

Whichever protein powder you choose, check the ingredients list for crap you don't want, like preservatives, excessive amounts of sugar, artificial sweeteners, or things you can't pronounce and suspect shouldn't really be going into your body.

HOW TO TELL "GOOD CARBS" FROM "BAD CARBS"

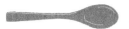

WHEN IT COMES to carbohydrates, we hear a lot about "good carbs" and "bad carbs." If you think this is confusing as hell, you're not alone. My clients complain that carb drama clouds their thinking and stresses them out.

To be honest, I hate using the words "good" and "bad" when it comes to food. This sets up a tricky dichotomy that can become a slippery slope for nagging feelings of guilt that drag you way down. We'll talk more about food guilt later, but if you've ever gone down a pasta/pizza/bread-induced shame spiral that took up way too much of your energy, you likely have an idea of what I'm talking about.

Here's what you need to know.

What Are Carbs, Anyway?
Carbohydrates are molecules that are comprised of carbon, hydrogen, and oxygen atoms. Most of the carbohydrates we eat are broken down by the digestive system into glucose, which is then used for energy to fuel our cells, tissues, and organs. Carbs can also be stored, so to speak, as fat cells for later use.

Carbs are made up of fiber, starch, and sugar. There are 4 calories per gram of carbohydrates. You'll often hear the terms "simple" carbs and "complex" carbs. Simple carbs are sugar—both the naturally occurring sugar present in foods and sugar that's added to sweeten them. Some common examples of simple carbs are sugar-sweetened beverages, candy, white flour products, and fruit juice.

Complex carbs are generally higher in fiber and digest more slowly. Some common examples are whole grains, beans and legumes, starchy vegetables, and whole fruit.

When we eat carbs, our blood glucose (aka blood sugar) rises. Consuming carbs with foods that contain protein and/or fat slows the rate at which that breakdown occurs, which helps maintain a more steady blood sugar level rather than causing a sharp spike and then crash. Fiber also helps slow that digestive process.

So What "Counts" as a Carb Serving?

A serving of carbohydrate is equivalent to about 15 grams. Here are a few examples of what that looks like:

- 1 slice of bread
- ⅓–½ cup of cooked grain (rice, pasta, oats, etc)
- ⅓–½ cup of cooked (or ¼ cup dry) beans, peas, or lentils
- ½ cup of cooked potatoes or corn
- ½ medium baked potato or sweet potato
- 1 cup of cooked pumpkin or winter squash

- 1 small apple or pear
- half of a 9-inch banana
- ¾-1 cup of berries
- ¼ cup of dried fruit
- ½ cup of fruit juice

Carbs and Our Mood

We often hear about carbohydrates in the context of blood sugar management, sports performance, and weight, but they also play an important role in our mental health. Have you ever noticed that you felt kind of down or depressed when you attempted a very low-carb diet? Or, on the other end of the spectrum, have you ever found yourself craving carbs when you're feeling down or struggling with seasonal affective disorder (SAD)? It's not about your lacking willpower or being "bad" for wanting to eat carbs—it's about your body wanting to maintain stable serotonin levels.

The way it works is that eating carbohydrates promotes insulin release, which boosts absorption of the amino acid tryptophan, a precursor to serotonin. That said, it's very easy to overdo it on carbs, especially when you reach for simple carbs (lots of the stuff on the Frenemies food list in the Hanger Management chapter) that you burn through quickly but that don't keep you full for very long. That's how you wind up with your fingers mysteriously grazing the bottom of an empty bag of chips that was totally full, like, five minutes ago.

Choosing the right carbs, however, can make all the difference.

What Makes a Carb a "Good Carb?"
When you hear someone talk about "good" carbs, chances are they're talking about complex carbs. This is going to be your whole grains, starchy vegetables, beans, pea, lentils, and whole fruit. Again, complex carbs tend to be higher in fiber and break down more slowly.

What's a "Bad Carb?"
Generally speaking, white flours, sugar-sweetened foods and beverages, and low-fiber snacks like potato chips are on the "bad carb" list. I would add fruit juice as well, especially if you're going to be drinking it on an empty stomach. Yes, juice provides lots of important vitamins and minerals, but because it provides all the sugar in that fruit with none of the fiber to slow digestion, it hits your bloodstream super quickly and sets you up for a blood sugar spike and dip.

Where Does Alcohol Fit In?
My clients and I talk a lot about how to fit in alcohol. While I never encourage starting to drink if you don't currently drink alcohol, I don't believe that you have to cut it out completely to be healthy. While the amount of carbohydrate in different types of alcohol varies, to help my clients make space for it, cutting out a serving of carbohydrate can be an easy option. For example, if you're out to dinner, instead of having bread, wine, and dessert, pick the two you want the most.

Here are some examples of how to fit in those slow-burning complex carbs through your day:

At Breakfast:

- Whole grain toast
- Oatmeal makes a great blank canvas for sweet and savory breakfast bowls
- Fruit can be used in smoothies, yogurt bowls, or as a topping for oats, cereal, or toast
- Roasted potatoes pair well with eggs and vegetables

At Lunch:

- Beans, peas, and lentils also add protein and fiber to soups and salads
- Whole wheat bread is a great complex carb swap for white bread

At Dinner:

- Whole wheat and bean- or lentil-based pasta can be bulked up with vegetables and protein
- Roasted or baked sweet potatoes pair well with protein and veggies
- Winter squash is a slightly less starchy alternative to potatoes

At Snacks:

- Whole grain crackers pair well with high-protein

toppings like nut butter, ricotta, and cottage cheese
- Fruit can be enjoyed on its own or with nuts, nut butter, yogurt, or cheese
- Dry-roasted edamame and chickpeas are convenient options that also provide a lot of protein and fiber

What if You Really Want a "Bad" Carb?

I'm a believer in honoring cravings. Ask yourself why you're craving that food. If it's a physical craving, is there something else that might satisfy that need? If it's an emotional craving, will that food really help?

If you're like, "Just shut up—I just want it because I want it," then I say listen to that. Have the thing you really want, and move on with your life. Sometimes denying ourselves what we really want can lead us to fixate and overeat subpar substitutes, setting ourselves up to still feel deprived and miserable.

Planning ahead can also help. For example, if you know you want to have a piece of cake or another simple-carb treat, cut out a carb serving elsewhere in your day. For example, remove a piece of bread to enjoy an open-faced sandwich with a side salad for a meal that's still satisfying but won't send you on a blood-sugar roller coaster.

HOW TO BREAK UP WITH ADDED SUGAR

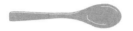

WE TALKED A little about sugar in the Frenemy Foods section of the Hanger Management chapter, and for good reason—it's one of those foods that wants you to think it's fun and awesome, but that can actually make you feel, well, pretty awful. For people who really struggle with feeling like they're addicted to sugar, it can even feel like an unhealthy codependent relationship.

There's no question that sugar isn't doing us any favors. Excess intake of sugar has been linked to weight gain and obesity as well as depressive symptoms and poor psychological health.[53] However, it's not just as simple as "eat less sugar." It's not always clear what types of sugar we should avoid and how to actually go about reducing our sugar intake in the context of a diet where we may not even be aware of all the different places it's coming from.

What's the Difference Between Natural and Added Sugar?

Naturally occurring sugar is the sugar that is naturally

present in foods: think fructose in fruit, lactose in dairy, glucose in starchy vegetables and grains. Even though natural sugar is natural, we don't want to overdo it. That said, because you're eating it as part of a whole food, other nutrients like fiber can help buffer the breakdown of that sugar.

Added sugars are sugars added to food to make it sweet. Just keep in mind that on a food label, you may see sugar listed under a wide variety of names. For example, anything with an "-ose" at the end. Maple syrup, brown rice syrup, cane sugar, and so on. While they certainly sound more natural, they still count as added sugar because they're being added. Stevia and other noncaloric sugar alternatives could also be considered added sweeteners, but we'll get to the reason I recommend limiting these too.

Added sugar is the type you want to keep to a minimum. While it adds taste and provides calories, it doesn't actually provide any vitamins, minerals, or other nutrients we need to function.

How Much Added Sugar Is Too Much?

Like all carbohydrates, one gram of sugar provides four calories. That may not sound like much, but over the course of a day, a week, all those tiny amounts can really add up. *The Dietary Guidelines for Americans*, which is developed by the U.S. Department of Health and Human Services (HHS) and Agriculture (USDA), recommends that adults limit added sugar to no more than 10 percent of their daily calorie intake—about 200 calories or 50 grams for someone on a 2,000-calorie diet. As a dietitian, that still sounds like a lot to me. That's more than 12 teaspoons!

The American Heart Association is a little more conservative, with its recommendation to cap added sugar at no more than 100 calories per day for women and 150 per day for men—so 6 or 9 teaspoons, respectively.[54]

Even then, less is still more. With sugar, the more you have, the more you tend to want. And, unfortunately, artificial sweeteners and sugar substitutes are not a sustainable workaround. While we may not have established which ones are the worst or exactly how bad for us they are, there hasn't exactly been any research showing that they're actively good for us or have health-promoting properties.

The main reason I discourage relying heavily on artificial sweeteners, though, is more psychological. While they may not have the caloric impact of sugar, they sidestep the underlying issue, which is dependence on and craving for sweetness. If we continue to condition ourselves to expect a high level of sweetness, how are we ever going to feel satisfied with foods that are naturally (and more mildly) sweet?

I went through a freaky experience in my mid-twenties when I decided to cut out diet soda. It started as an experiment—all I did was switch to seltzer for a few weeks. What I soon found, though, was that I could no longer stand the pink packets I used to add to my coffee. Flavored yogurts started tasting way too sweet. Baked goods made me sick to my stomach. As someone who was used to wanting to eat dessert and all manner of sugar-free crap, it was baffling—it was like my sweet tooth had fallen out. Had my heavy-duty artificial sweetener use been behind it all along? I didn't even need to know the answer; I just felt so much better that I never wanted to go back.

So How Do I Break Up with Sugar?

There are a few different ways to reduce your intake of added sugar. You can make a clean break and cut out all forms of added sugar, or you can do the slow fade. Some people will want to get super strict about it, whereas others may choose to draw the line in a different place. Here are some steps to follow.

- **Identify where the added sugar in your diet comes from**. A piece of cake on your birthday or a planned-for holiday treat is one thing—sugar creeping into your yogurt or your cereal, not to mention pasta sauce, marinades, frozen meals, and wholesome-sounding snacks is a whole other ball game. That's not playing fair; that's just sneaky.
- **Get real with yourself about how much of it you're eating**. I know I threw some numbers at you earlier as a ballpark figure, but you're the expert on you. Do you feel like your sugar intake is in a realistic place, or do you want it to be lower?
- **Decide where to draw the line**. Be honest with yourself about what you can and can't be moderate with.

Some people can have five M&Ms and then put the bag away. Other people have to finish the whole thing.

- **Take sugar off the pedestal**. This one is easier said than done, but practice telling yourself that it's just a food. That sugar is just a molecule. Wanting or eating it does not make you good or bad—and if you make a choice that doesn't support your goal, forgive yourself and move on. Resist the "I've blown it" mind-set and focus instead on what choices will help restore some balance and positivity to your day.

- **Educate yourself**. Read labels, check ingredients. Scope out other options and keep track of what you like that suits your needs and preferences.

- **Find new favorites**. Rather than focus on restriction, look at this as an opportunity to try new things and experiment. For example, try out some new products and recipes that provide lots of flavor without added sugar.

- **Make it easy**. If you're trying to reduce your sugar intake, get it out of your house. If you know that going cold turkey is just not going to work for you, then gradually step it down. You can focus on cutting out one source at a time or try going halfsies on sweetened and unsweetened versions of products like yogurt and cereal. Shift the ratio as your taste buds adjust over time. Another approach is to gradually decrease the number of sugar or sweetener packets you use in your coffee.

Choose Your Moments

Have sugar when you truly want it. Enjoy and then move on. Know what you can and can't be moderate about. Resist the urge to judge yourself. When you make room for what you truly love by skipping the stuff you don't, it can help you feel satisfied and keep you on track for the long haul.

THE OVERTHINK-PROOF PLATE

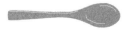

PORTION SIZES CAN be daunting. We hear all this stuff about cups and grams and tablespoons and macronutrients, and it's enough to make your head spin. To help simplify your life and give you flexibility in any dining situation, follow this overthink-proof formula for at least two meals per day:

THE OVERTHINK-PROOF PLATE

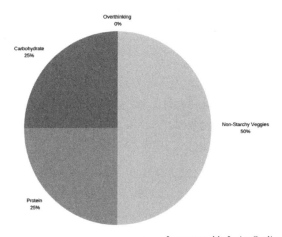

Image created by Jessica Cording

Fill half your plate with non-starchy veggies. In that category, you've got stuff like:

- leafy greens
- asparagus
- cruciferous vegetables, including broccoli, cauliflower, and brussels sprouts
- cucumber
- eggplant
- peppers
- zucchini and summer squash

Fill a quarter of your plate with protein, which could be animal or plant protein. A few examples:

- meat
- poultry
- fish
- eggs
- dairy
- beans, lentils
- nuts, seeds, or nut or seed butter
- tofu, tempeh, or other soy product
- seitan (made from vital wheat gluten)

Fill the last quarter of your plate with carbohydrates, which could include:

- Grains
- Starchy vegetables like potato, sweet potato, winter squash, corn, or peas
- Beans or lentils (if they're not serving as your protein source)
- Fruit

Here are a few examples of what a full meal might look like, whether you're using a plate, bowl, or glass:

- Two eggs with a half cup of roasted sweet potato and 1 cup of sautéed greens
- A piece of cooked meat, fish, or tofu with 1 cup of broccoli and a half cup of brown rice or quinoa
- A green smoothie made with plain Greek yogurt, half a frozen banana, half a cup of frozen berries, and 2 cups of baby spinach

If you're wondering where fat fits in, I'm glad you asked. As a rule of thumb, aim to have a source of fat at each of your meals, whether that's in cooking oil, a garnish of nuts or cheese, or avocado or a spread like guacamole or hummus.

Also, if you're someone who prefers to eat a sweet breakfast or are wondering what to do about snacks, aim to have a balance of protein, fat, and carbs and just make sure you cover your bases with vegetables later in the day.

FIND YOUR SWEET SPOT
WITH CAFFEINE

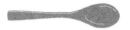

IF YOU HAVE a mug, T-shirt, or tattoo that says something like, "But first, coffee," you're in good company. My relationship with this legal addictive stimulant is the longest romantic relationship in my life—so far, anyway. I've had to learn the hard way, though, that too much of a good thing is possible. Sound familiar? Then this chapter on finding your sweet spot with caffeine is for you.

My love affair with coffee started when I was very young, sneaking sips of my mother's deli coffee with half-and-half in it. By the time I was in high school, I couldn't start my morning without caffeine. My tastes and preferences morphed and evolved over the years, but by the time I was in my mid-twenties I was drinking about eight cups of black coffee a day—at least on the days I was working at the hospital, where the Starbucks counter was a welcome refuge from the crowded nutrition office. I'd start with a 24-ounce cup while I was getting ready for work in the morning, another 16 ounces during morning rounds, and then usually another 16 ounces in the afternoon when I took a walk around the block.

The winter I was thirty, though, my insomnia was the worst it had been in years. I would wake up at 3 a.m. many nights, unable to sleep. I got into this strange routine where I'd go tire myself out doing thirty minutes of cardio in my building's basement gym, take a shower, and go back to bed. I chalked it up to work stress. Those heart palpitations? Anxiety. Feeling sad about my love life—anything but coffee.

I finally decided to see my doctor, who asked me a bunch of questions about what was going on in my life and then finally got to, "So how much coffee are you drinking?"

Yeah. That.

So, Wait, Is Caffeine Good or Bad?

Coffee (caffeine, in general) actually has been shown to have some health benefits, but how much we consume and when we consume it plays a big role. According to the 2015-2020 *Dietary Guidelines for Americans*, a healthy adult can safely consume up to 400 milligrams of caffeine per day, which is equivalent to about four 8-ounce cups of brewed coffee per day, unless you're drinking a stronger cup, such as Starbucks, where a Grande of drip coffee can clock in anywhere from 260-360 milligrams, depending on the type you get.[55]

A shot of espresso has about 75 milligrams of caffeine and tea also provides caffeine, depending on the type and steeping duration. According to the Mayo Clinic, black tea, for example, contains anywhere from 14 to 70 milligrams per cup, and green tea has 24 to 45 milligrams.[56]

Regular coffee intake has been linked to improved short-term memory function and a lower risk of diabetes, certain cancers, cognitive decline, and neurological conditions like Alzheimer's disease. A small to moderate dose (20–200 milligrams or one to two cups) has been shown to improve exercise endurance. There's also the social component to consider. Connecting with friends, family, and colleagues over a cup of coffee or tea is a central part of many cultures.

However, caffeine may not be appropriate for people with certain heart conditions, and excess intake can lead to sleep disturbances, gastrointestinal discomfort, and it may also amp up anxiety. Of course, there's also caffeine withdrawal, where you experience headaches, irritability, and even flu-like symptoms when you don't get your fix. Another big one is that coffee and tea beverages can easily become vehicles for sugar, which can contribute a lot of excess calories that may not actually feel like anything.

Some people are more sensitive to caffeine than others. Many factors can impact how the body metabolizes caffeine. A few big ones are smoking, some medical conditions, and the use of certain medications, such as oral contraceptives. A person's sweet spot with caffeine—namely, how much they can consume without feeling negative effects—can vary greatly between individuals, and it can change over time as they go through changes.

How Do You Cut Back on Caffeine Without Going Crazy?

If you suspect your caffeine intake is way above your sweet spot, there's hope. If it's not realistic (or medically necessary) for you to quit cold turkey or sharply reduce your intake right away, a gradual approach can help you get to where you want to be with a minimum of pain.

- **Set a clear goal.** Rather than vowing to "cut back," get specific with yourself. What is your ideal amount of caffeine? How far are you from that? How long do you want to take to get to your goal? Say you want to go from six cups a day to one—you could start by having five cups a day for a week or two, four cups a day for the next week or two, and so on until you reach your goal.

- **Identify barriers.** Take an honest look at the role caffeine plays in your life, and be real about situations where you might be tempted to revert back to old habits. For example, there might be that "need" piece where you feel like crap when you don't have a cup in the morning, or it's your little bit of "me" time before the rest of your household wakes up for the day. Maybe taking a walk to go get a cup of coffee in the middle of your workday can be the only way you feel like you can take a break, or helps you reach your steps goal. Or maybe that cup of coffee with a friend is an important part of your social life.

- **Be prepared.** Now that you've identified which situations you may need a plan for, you can brainstorm some ways to work through those barriers. You could start by changing your order from a large to a small (or switching to a smaller mug at home or at the office), or by cutting it with half-decaf. You might also consider a non-coffee beverage like green or herbal tea, or even water or seltzer. This can actually be a great time to branch out and try new things. Remind yourself that it's about the experience more than anything.

  That said, if physical dependency is your issue, be realistic about the fact that you'll probably have some withdrawal symptoms. While gradually reducing your caffeine intake does help guard against this, your body's not stupid—it will usually notice if you make a change like that. Remind yourself that your headache, irritability, and other symptoms are temporary and will get better. However, if it helps you manage your energy through the day, make note of when you tend to suffer most and plan to do tasks that require less focus or interaction with others. If possible, give yourself a few breaks through the day.

- **Set a curfew**. Because caffeine can impact us for many hours after we drink it, setting a time to cut yourself off can help avoid caffeine-related sleep disturbances.

- **Prioritize nutrition**. A really common thing I see with clients who are cutting back on caffeine is cravings for sugar or fatty, nutrient-dense foods. Rather than try to white-knuckle it and ignore those cravings, acknowledge them and make sure to fuel yourself with well-balanced meals and snacks that provide a stabilizing balance of protein, fat, and carbs. Drink plenty of water too—even mild dehydration can make you feel sluggish, exacerbating withdrawal symptoms.

- **Be active**. Endorphins are magic for boosting energy and mood when you're feeling droopy. If a formal workout or gym visit just doesn't feel like an option, a brisk walk or other gentle movement you enjoy totally counts.

- **Establish a solid sleep routine**. This is a great time to get into a consistent routine with your sleep and wake times. Aim to go to bed and wake up within an hour or two of the same time each day—yes, even on weekends. Having morning and evening rituals you enjoy (as we talked about in the chapter on embracing routine) can make this process feel like good self-care rather than a chore.

Bottom Line

Caffeine may have some health benefits when consumed in moderation, but having too much can cause problems. Creating a plan to help you gradually get to your sweet spot can help you enjoy it without feeling like a slave to it.

THE POWER OF A
FOOD-MOOD JOURNAL

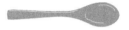

A FOOD JOURNAL is one of the most-used diet tools. Whether you're using a pen and paper, a document on your computer, or an app, tracking what you eat and drink can provide useful insight into your eating habits and help you spot patterns and potential gaps you need to address. The "what" we put in our mouths is only part of the picture, though. I encourage all my clients to keep a food-mood journal to help them dig into the "why" behind their choices.

What Is a Food-Mood Journal?

A food-mood journal is basically what it sounds like. You log what you eat, but also write down how you felt emotionally before, during, and/or after that eating occasion. You may find it helpful to also note things like what the environment or situation was like and whom you were with. The overall purpose of this journal is to help you identify links between your emotions and your eating habits.

Why Does It Work?

Often, even though we're aware of *what* we're eating, we may be overlooking the emotional or psychological factors that cause us to make choices that don't support our goals. Sometimes you know if you're an emotional overeater (or under-eater, which is also a thing). But not infrequently, I see people who are completely convinced that their eating isn't tied to their emotions come to realize that how they're feeling actually plays a huge role.

Honestly, I think that on some level we all experience a degree of this in our life. Learning to see the connections between our emotions and our eating patterns can help us identify the changes we can make. For example, you may notice you always want to stop for ice cream after your dinners with that friend who triggers your compar-itis, or that you have a hard time resisting donuts at your Thursday morning team meetings. Maybe you've found that when you're feeling triggered by current events or under pressure to meet a work deadline, you're too nauseous to eat and wind up with energy crashes and hanger-induced meltdowns.

Knowing these things about yourself can lead you to make changes, such as going to the movies instead of coffee chats with that friend, or bringing your breakfast to that meeting so you won't be tempted by the donuts. Finding ways to deal with stressors that kill your appetite, such as talking to a therapist or coming up with a system to make projects less overwhelming, can make a big difference.

How to Keep a Food-Mood Journal

There are many ways to keep a food-mood journal. Whether you're keeping a hard or electronic copy, you can be as loose or as thorough as you find helpful. For someone who's just getting into a groove with this, I recommend being a little more detailed and consistent than someone who's been practicing this for a long time and has a pretty good handle on what sets them off and how to reroute when they need to.

Here's a basic format to get you started:

- Write down the time
- What the meal or snack was (breakfast, morning snack, etc.)
- What the meal or snack consisted of
- Where you were eating
- Anyone else you were eating with
- Emotions before eating (this can include thoughts, feelings, stress level, etc.)
- Emotions during the meal
- Emotions after the meal
- If desired, any physical sensations before, during, or after the meal

If this sounds like a lot, I promise it becomes much more automatic over time. For many people, they get to a place where they don't feel a need to keep a daily log but keep the food-mood journal in their back pocket as a useful tool for when they feel like they're going through a stressful time and prone to getting off track.

HOW TO TURN MEALTIMES INTO A CHANCE TO DE-STRESS

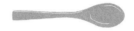

CONFESSION: AS A teenager, I ate most of my meals either in the car or standing up at a shelf I used as a desk while I did homework. We had family dinners on the weekends or went out sometimes, but I was on my own a lot of the time and didn't really see any point in stopping what I was doing. When I went to college, I lived on campus for the first two years and ate in the dining hall, but when I moved into my first apartment, I ate most of my meals sitting on the floor in front of my laptop while I wrote. When I finally got a table that wasn't a coffee table, of course I turned it into a make-shift desk.

It really wasn't until I moved to New York and into an apartment with a boyfriend that the concept of a table you use just for eating and not as your office started to make sense. Oh, right—connecting with another person over a meal. So *that's* what all the fuss was about. That said, most of our fights took place over that same table, so I also got a taste of what it's like when dinner becomes a high-anxiety part of your day.

While I managed to avoid turning that table into my workspace after he moved out, I gradually slid back into my old habit of eating at my desk while working. Then when I started working in a hospital that had no cafeteria, I started eating lunch while catching up on patient notes so that I could use my lunch break to take a walk instead of trying to go find a place to sit. Since I worked the early shift, I usually ate breakfast at my desk while I screened patients before morning rounds.

No wonder I felt like I never got a break! I was eating two to three meals a day in front of a screen.

I definitely noticed a difference in how satisfied I felt after eating when I allowed myself to slow down and get away from the machines. It's hardly news that "distracted eating" can dampen our perception of satisfaction, making it all too easy to plow through larger portions than we need. If you're cooking for and serving yourself and paying attention to serving size at home, or eating a packed lunch, it's less of an issue in the short-term, but it can feel damn near impossible to stay on track when you're wolfing down takeout, finding your way to the bottom of a bag of chips, or your brown-bag lunch barely holds you over an hour before you start looking for snacks in the break room.

And besides, when we don't give ourselves breaks in our day to sit and eat and mentally recharge, whatever is stressing us out and making us anxious just keeps gnawing at us all day. Having gone through this struggle myself (and let's be real—I still go through phases where I have a hard time taking a break), I've come up with some simple hacks to help my clients reclaim mealtimes and turn them into a chance to dial down stress.

- **Clear a place to sit and eat**. I know this one can be hard, but it's so important. If tearing yourself away for a lunch break feels impossible, remind yourself that stopping—even if it's only for fifteen minutes—will give you more energy to tackle whatever tasks you're working on that afternoon. I understand that some workplaces may not be conducive to eating anywhere other than your desk (been there!), so designate a space by moving around papers and facing away from your computer, if possible. At home, get your ass up off the couch or from your computer chair and sit at the table where you eat meals, or if you don't have a table, turn off the screen or pause what you're watching. This is often the hardest part!
- **Use real plates and silverware**. Even if you're eating a frozen meal or takeout, the thirty seconds it takes to put your food on an actual plate and trade the plastic cutlery for the real stuff can majorly upgrade your eating experience.
- **Minimize distractions**. Many of us are used to eating with our phone on the table or the TV blaring. We might be so used to it we don't even realize how much those things impact us. So turn off the set and keep your phone away from the table (if you're

someone who routinely takes a picture of your food, fine, but take the photo and then put your phone out of reach). You can post onto social media after you eat. If the phone rings, you really don't have to answer it. You could also try putting your phone into Do Not Disturb mode, and if you're worried about missing a call, adjust your settings so the people you want to be available to will still get through.

And if sitting in silence is just too weird for you, try playing soft music or listening to an audiobook or podcast.

- **Slow down.** This is one of my favorite hacks: put your fork down between bites. It's an easy way to pace yourself and avoid overeating.

- **Set the mood**. Even when you're dining alone, you want to create a comfortable environment. Turn off harsh overhead lights in favor of softer lighting from lamps (or consider a dimmer switch). Light candles if you want to. It might seem cheesy the first few times you do it—especially if you're eating alone—but you'll likely come to find you really enjoy it.

Dining with a partner or family members can have both positive and negative impacts on your meals. It's not uncommon to notice changes in our eating habits when we're with others, and as I mentioned above, sometimes conversations that come up around the table may not always be pleasant.

- **Practice mindful serving**. Many of my clients say that they find it harder to stick to appropriate portion sizes if others at their table are eating more. If that sounds familiar, one thing that can help is plating your meal at the counter and leaving any serving containers there, or even putting them in the fridge, so that if you do want seconds, you have to commit to getting up for it. Many people find they may eat more or less depending on whom they're dining with, so pay attention to see if you notice any patterns.
- **Plan if you need to.** When you're eating with someone who follows a very different diet from you (for example, one partner is vegan but the other is not, or one family member has an allergy or intolerance), navigating what to eat can become stressful and/or anxiety provoking. A little advance planning can go a long way toward tempering that drama in the moment.

  If you're worried about conversations taking a stressful turn, consider making certain topics off-limits over dinner. For example, put a hold on talking about work drama, or set aside time for to-do-list chatter so you don't feel like you spend the whole meal filling your brain with more stuff you have to do.

  Be patient with yourself and others. Sometimes simply taking a deep breath can help you let go of whatever drama you showed up with.

5 WAYS TO CREATE A MEAL PLAN YOU CAN STICK TO

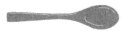

WHEN I WAS a new dietitian, I used to pour *so* much energy into creating intricate plans detailing what my clients should eat for breakfast, lunch, dinner, and snacks seven days a week, complete with recipes. That was what I'd learned in school, and one of the first things people always asked when finding out my profession was, "So can you make me a meal plan?"

Hell yeah, I could.

Here's the thing, though—a meal plan is effective only when you're actually able to follow it.

More often than not I would hear, "I tried, but I got too busy to cook" or "My in-laws were in town and we went out every night" or "I had chips one day and then was like, 'Well, I already blew it, so . . .'" or "It turned out to be a really stressful week and I just wanted to eat comfort food."

In theory, the meal plans were awesome, but when my clients' plans for the week changed and they didn't feel prepared to think on the fly, they found it easier to revert to their old unhealthy habits. Sure, they had a plan, but that plan didn't account for their real life and the madness that often ensues and throws all kinds of curveballs at us.

It didn't take long for me to change my approach. While I'll still give recipes to clients who want them and will give specific suggestions for meals and snacks, the actual meal plans I create are way more flexible, usually focusing more on having a balance of protein, veggies, fat, and carbs and keeping an eye on portion size and timing, so my clients stay satisfied and energized. I want my clients to know they can navigate those tricky days when plans change and roll with the punches without feeling like they're on a diet they go on and off of.

Here are five ways to create a meal plan you can actually stick to.

1. Factor in Your Schedule
Take five or ten minutes over the weekend (or whatever day works for your schedule) to look over what you have coming up in the week ahead to get a sense of when you'll be eating at home and when you might be dining out or having to figure out meals or snacks on the go.

2. Keep It Loose
Look at food groups instead of exact recipes. The idea is that you want to feel like that formula of filling half your plate (or bowl) with veggies, a quarter with protein, and a quarter with carbs can give you freedom to choose what you're in

the mood for or work with what's available if you're in a situation with limited options.

3. Play Favorites

Keeping track of favorite recipes in a file or a Pinterest board where you can easily find them can save you a ton of time when figuring out what to make for the week ahead. I also encourage my clients to keep a list of their favorite healthy takeout, restaurants, and grab-and-go items to reduce decision-making fatigue when they're in a rush or feeling stressed out. You can keep a mental list or even a physical or electronic one. Many years ago, in one of my past lives as a PR intern, I had a boss who kept a few go-to lunch orders in a folder in an electronic file. That was so brilliant! It saved time and reduced the chances of my screwing up the order.

4. Make It a Joint Effort

If you're coordinating with your partner, family, or roommates, making meal planning a joint effort can make the process so much easier. While you could sit down together once a week and talk through what everyone wants to have, if that's not realistic, a family Google Doc everyone can add to or an app that lets you share documents and lists can streamline the process. It's also a great way to share shopping lists.

5. Learn from Your Mistakes

Whether it's with food or something else, we've all been in situations where we set a plan but just couldn't seem to stick with it. Rather than blame yourself or your lack of willpower, think about what, specifically, was so challenging. This may give you clues as to what sorts of tweaks will help you going forward.

MEAL PREP HACKS TO STREAMLINE YOUR COOKING

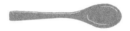

PREPARING FOOD AHEAD of time can be a major game changer. Having ingredients washed, chopped, and cooked makes it so much easier to assemble healthy meals when you're short on time or trying to stick to a budget.

When we think about meal prep in the social media #mealprep sense of the word, we tend to think of elaborate spreads of identical pre-portioned meals, meant to be toted to the office. We also are conditioned to think that this prep has to happen on Sundays and that it must take a lot of time and effort. And that it must look pretty.

Honestly, though, you could microwave a bag of frozen broccoli on a Tuesday night and that still counts as meal prep if it's giving you an ingredient that you can use in future meals, simplifying your life and making it easier to eat well.

And yes, even if you work from home, as more and more people do, meal prep can still be helpful for you. Ever notice how hard it is to regain momentum in the afternoon if you pause to prepare and eat lunch? While a lunch break is important, you don't have to derail your productivity by cooking from scratch every day.

You could also call it batch cooking, where you make big batches of vegetables, proteins, and carbs. I also like to think of it sometimes as turning your fridge into a salad or stir-fry bar.

Here are some of my favorite meal prep hacks that can streamline your cooking:

- Keep a few containers of washed and trimmed greens on hand. You can use them as salad bases, and some of the heartier ones like kale, spinach, and arugula can also work in cooked dishes. You just might want to zap them in the microwave if you're in a hurry.
- Chop up some of your favorite veggies (a few I love are brussels sprouts, broccoli, cauliflower, and asparagus), toss them with olive oil, and roast them on a sheet pan until they're soft and starting to get crispy. This gives you some great options to throw into salads, grain bowls, omelets, and frittatas. They're also just great side dish options.
- While you've got the oven turned on, you can bake some chicken, tofu, or a batch of meatballs or egg muffins.
- Your slow cooker or instant pot is your best friend for preparing a big batch of a protein like chicken or pork, beans, or a hearty soup, stew, or chili.

- Hard-boiled eggs are another great protein option that don't require much hands-on work.
- If you're a fan of spiralized vegetables, make a large batch so you can just grab what you need when you're ready for it.
- A big pot of whole grains, lentils, or chickpeas can be stretched and repurposed in all kinds of ways throughout the week.
- Don't forget accents. A few of my favorites that keep for a few days in the fridge are caramelized onions and mushroom bacon (basically, sliced mushrooms tossed with olive oil, a little maple syrup, and savory spices, and baked until crispy and delicious). If you enjoy cheese as a garnish, you can grate your favorite and keep it in an airtight container in the fridge, using just a little at a time. You can also make your own salad dressing and keep it refrigerated for up to a week.

Some other hacks to simplify your life:

- Stock frozen produce. Keeping frozen vegetables and fruit handy can cut down on food waste, and it also makes it easy to always have healthy bases for meals and snacks around if you travel a lot or have an inconsistent schedule that makes it hard to know how much fresh produce to buy. I also love it because if you're purchasing organic, it's generally much easier to find what you want in your budget no matter the season. Also, because these foods are frozen at peak freshness, it locks in all that nutritious goodness so you can reap the benefits.

- Use meal kits. There are so many great options on the market now where you can choose the number of healthy recipes you want for the week, and you'll get a box with the ingredients you need—so much easier than trying to figure it out on your own! Sometimes these kits tend to be a little grain- and meat-heavy, so just know you may want to supplement with extra veggies. This can also help you stretch the portions an extra meal or two.

- Do mini-meal preps. If you feel that carving out a few solid hours to prep food isn't a reality, you can totally split your meal prep into a few mini sessions. Like I said, a half hour on a Tuesday totally counts.

Whatever approach you take, remember that the goal is to simplify. If you find that meal prep stresses you out or overwhelms you, give yourself permission to dial it back a little. Trying out different recipes or even just using different seasonings to prepare your staples can help if you're worried about getting bored. And make sure you're cooking food you love and look forward to eating.

HEALTHY SNACK HACKS

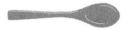

SNACKING GETS A bad reputation, but when you're on the go or have long stretches between meals, it can be a useful way to keep your energy up and prevent overeating when you finally get around to sitting down for a meal. For example, if lunch is at noon and dinner doesn't happen until 8 p.m., it's completely reasonable (and smart) to eat something in the afternoon.

Snacking can also be useful for helping us manage our stress and anxiety because it supports stable blood sugar levels. This is key for helping us think clearly so we can handle it when stuff comes up, and it helps us avoid those "hangry" meltdowns when we have low blood sugar and feel like we just can't deal with the crazy at hand. Snacks also offer a good opportunity to work in stress-busting superfoods such as antioxidant-rich berries, brain-soothing monounsaturated fats in avocados and olive oil, and dopamine (aka pleasure chemical)-boosting folate in oranges. And that's just to name a few!

There are no set-in-stone rules for snacking, but, in

general, I encourage you to grab a quick bite if you've got a stretch longer than four hours between meals or, of course, when you're legitimately hungry. On a scale of 1 to 10, with 1 being so hungry you feel light-headed and 10 being absolutely stuffed, eat when you're at or below 3.

As for what to eat, as a (very) general guideline, I recommend keeping snacks to about 100-250 calories and choosing something that provides a balance of protein and fiber. Aim for at least 5 grams of protein and 3 grams of fiber, and keep added sugar as low as possible—ideally less than 5 grams.

To briefly recap what I talked about in the chapter on sugar, naturally occurring sugar is a sugar (aka carbohydrate) that is naturally present in a food—think fructose in fruit and glucose in grains. Added sugars, on the other hand, are added to a food to make it sweet. This may include white sugar, but it also applies to things like honey, brown rice syrup, evaporated cane juice, maltodextrin, and the many other names we may see for sugar on a food label.

You're probably sick of hearing this, but whole foods without added ingredients (like sweeteners) help you enjoy the most nutritional bang for your buck without tacking on a bunch of crap you don't need.

That doesn't mean you have to get precious about it or spend hours preparing food.

Here are some easy snack ideas:

Sweet

- Berries and plain Greek yogurt or cottage cheese
- DIY trail mix (a quarter cup nuts or seeds and 1 tablespoon dried fruit)
- 1 small sweet potato steamed in the microwave and topped with 1 tablespoon of unsweetened nut butter
- 1 slice whole grain toast topped with 2 tablespoons ricotta cheese and berries (for a savory twist, use sliced tomatoes or leftover roasted vegetables)

Savory

- half a cup of hummus or guacamole and sliced vegetables
- 2 hard-boiled eggs and sliced vegetables
- 1 ounce cheese with whole grain crackers
- 1 cup of broth-based vegetable soup with beans or meat
- Half an avocado with one tablespoon of hemp hearts

What to Stuff Your Face with when Stress Snacking Is Inevitable

Stress-snacking can put a huge dent in your self-confidence—not just your diet. While I work with my clients to find strategies for establishing healthy responses when they want to stress-eat, it's an inevitable thing for many people, so having a few go-to options in your back pocket can minimize the damage. The top stress-eating foods I recommend are:

- **Blueberries**—Blueberries are packed with filling fiber and key vitamins and minerals. Plus, the antioxidants in blueberries have been shown to benefit brain function and stress response. A serving is also a full cup.
- **Popcorn**—When you want something crunchy or want to be able to eat a huge serving of something, popcorn is a great pick. A serving is about 3 cups, which will only set you back about 100 calories. This whole grain also provides around 3 grams each of fiber and protein per serving, so it will actually help satisfy you. Just be mindful that add-ons like butter, caramel, and the like will contribute excess calories that could end up negating those benefits. Keep it simple with an air-popped variety and toss it with your favorite spices if you need more flavor.
- **Oranges**—Aside from its cheerful color and bright citrus taste, oranges are also a great source of folate, a nutrient that's key to supporting efficient production of dopamine, a brain chemical that's associated with how we experience pleasure. Plus, the act of peeling an orange gives your hands something to do.
- **Pistachios**—Pistachios contain filling fiber and heart-healthy fats, which also benefit the brain. The main reason they get my stress-eating pick, though, is because a serving is 45 pistachios, which is double the recommended serving of almonds (22). Shelling them yourself can be very soothing to the mind and occupies your hands so you don't reach for other stuff.

DO I REALLY NEED
TO EAT BREAKFAST?

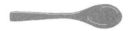

SOME PEOPLE LOVE breakfast, some people hate it, but pretty much all of us have grown up being told it's the most important meal of the day. But is it really?

Spoiler alert: I do tend to encourage eating something within the first couple hours of waking, but it doesn't have to be anything big or elaborate. You need to let your body be your guide.

As a kid, I was always baffled by the "balanced breakfast" I saw in commercials. The idea of pairing a bowl of cereal with a side of toast as well as juice just seemed weird (something about the sweet-savory-sour combo didn't add up in my brain), but to someone else, that may have seemed totally normal. You want to talk about weird, though? I went through a phase in high school where I was all about soup for breakfast and meatballs in marinara sauce as an after-school snack—salty foods to match a salty personality, I guess. Like many teenagers, I was just a little blue ball of fire at seventeen.

Anyway, my teen and college years were actually the

beginning of my interest in the connection between what we eat and how we feel mentally and how efficiently we perform in our work. I noticed how much better my day went when I had a balanced morning meal than if I tried to dive in on just an apple, a piece of leftover Halloween candy, and a 20-ounce Diet Mountain Dew downed on the way to class. I don't know what I was thinking, but like I said, teenagers and college kids are, like, another species. For whatever reason, it's a necessary part of human evolution!

When clients ask me if breakfast is really important, here's what I tell them.

Why You Should Eat Breakfast

I'm a firm believer in the idea that how we start our day sets the tone for what's to come. That doesn't mean that if you have a rough morning you can't get back into a positive groove, but nourishing your body can certainly give you a leg up.

A morning meal that provides you with a combination of protein and complex carbs gives you stable blood sugar so you'll have the energy you need to power through your to-do list and keep those hangry meltdowns away. Eating breakfast can also help prevent overeating when you finally get to lunch.

Having breakfast can also serve as a grounding ritual before you get into your day. Even a few moments to focus on the smell and taste of what you're eating can get you into a calmer mind-set. No matter what the day has in store, you've done something kind for yourself.

Lack of time is one of the main reasons breakfast falls by the wayside for a lot of people, so here are a few easy breakfast combos for busy days:

- A piece of fruit and nut butter
- A latte or cappuccino and a serving of nuts, seeds, or an egg
- A hard-boiled egg and a piece of fruit
- Oats with nut butter
- A slice of whole grain toast with an egg or nut butter
- Plain Greek yogurt with fruit

If you're a fan of morning workouts or have the kind of schedule where you may need to get up early but don't actually have the opportunity to sit down to a full meal until later in the morning, you can also split your morning into Breakfast Part 1 and Breakfast Part 2.

Why You Might Not Need Breakfast

If you're not hungry in the morning, that doesn't mean you're a bad person or there's something wrong with you. And if the thought of eating first thing makes you want to hurl, then don't force it.

If you notice that you can't make it through the morning without snacking or that you overeat at lunch, you might want to consider starting your day with something small like a piece of fruit, a hard-boiled egg, or even a latte or cappuccino made with cow's milk or pea protein milk.

Bottom Line

You're the expert on you, so tune into what feels good in the morning. While breakfast is strongly encouraged, by no means is it necessary.

HEALTHIER LUNCH, MADE EASY

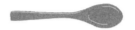

A HEALTHY LUNCH can make your afternoon much more enjoyable and productive. Many people find that it's hard to make it a regular habit, though. A few of the main reasons my clients share are feeling like they don't have enough time to make lunch or feeling like they shift into autopilot mode and reach for unhealthy comfort foods after a stressful morning when they've been working hard and have decision-making fatigue.

Here are a few of the game-changing tips that will help make it easier to enjoy a healthy lunch, especially if you're eating outside of your home.

Meal prep

Making sure to have some healthy foods you enjoy on hand makes it easier to assemble them into balanced meals throughout the week. You can batch-cook ingredients to throw together or assemble into different meals.

Pack lunch while you make dinner the night before

It sounds so simple but it's very powerful. As you plate your dinner, put leftovers into a to-go container for the next day. One of my favorite hacks is to put leftover meat and vegetables over greens. You could also repurpose stir-fry or use cooked protein in a sandwich.

Buy lunch at the beginning of the day

Some stores, delis, and cafes sell lunch foods starting early in the morning, so if grabbing what you know you need for lunch on your way to work early in the day cuts down on the chaos in the brain that sets in around noon, do it. It doesn't have to be crazy-early, either. You could go buy lunch around 11 a.m., just before the rush, even if you don't intend to eat for another few hours. Just make sure you store your food properly to avoid spoilage!

Keep track of your favorite takeout and grab-and-go options

Knowing what makes you feel nourished and satisfied is a good starting place for building a list of go-to lunch options. You can keep a mental list or make an actual list on your phone or computer. This will save you time and mental energy later.

WHAT TO EAT (AND AVOID)
FOR A GOOD NIGHT'S SLEEP

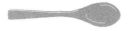

YOU DON'T NEED me to tell you that sleep is important. It's the top self-care non-negotiable of some of the most successful people in the world, and you yourself have likely noticed how much better and more effective you feel when you get enough quality rest than when you're short on shut-eye.

Sleep deprivation has been linked to many health problems, such as impaired cognitive function high blood pressure and increased risk of heart disease, diabetes, and obesity. The weight gain association that has been attributed to lack of sleep is due to changes in "hunger hormones" leptin and ghrelin, which lead us to feel sensations of hunger more strongly but to be less perceptive to those inner cues that tell us when we're satisfied (this tends to go hand in hand with a preference for sugary and fatty foods)—in short, it's a recipe for overeating. Sleep deprivation can also be dangerous—your risk of accident or injury goes way up when you're running on fumes.

So, yeah, sleep is a big deal. It's estimated that adults, on average, need about seven hours per night, and yet, so many of us struggle to clock that amount. A poor night of sleep here or there is one thing, but it can become a problem when inadequate quality sleep becomes a regular occurrence and sleep deprivation becomes someone's norm, as it is for many people (the CDC estimates that around 35 percent of adults report short sleep duration).[57]

There's a wide range of factors that can affect our sleep. Among the biggest are stress, anxiety, the sleep environment (things like temperature, light, and sound), medications, and even what and how much we eat and drink in the hours before bed.

For example, downing an espresso right before bed might keep you up. Or if you go to bed after eating a huge meal— or on the flip, side, really hungry—you may have trouble drifting off. Finding that sweet spot between starving and stuffed is key.

Specific foods can also play a part in helping you fall asleep and stay asleep thanks to the different nutrients and compounds they provide. Here are some of the main ones:

Melatonin[58]

This hormone regulates our circadian rhythm. Our levels increase in the dark, so pulling those shades down and blocking sources of light in your sleeping area are a good first step. While melatonin isn't present in many foods, supplements can be an easy way to work it in when you need it. That said, I wouldn't recommend it as a daily thing. It's not going to knock you out but is helpful for bringing your circadian rhythm back into a stable pattern when it goes out of whack. Ideally, you want to take melatonin for no more than a week at a time to help you when you're dealing with an inconsistent sleep schedule, traveling across time zones, or adjusting to seasonal time changes or changes in daylight hours.

Serotonin[59]

This mood-regulating neurotransmitter also regulates our sleep cycle by playing a role in that process of calming down so we can drift off. Serotonin is also involved in melatonin production. It's not found in many foods, but making sure we eat a variety of foods that support and enhance its production can help us maintain good levels. We'll get more into that later in this chapter.

Tryptophan[60]

Tryptophan is an amino acid that is a precursor to serotonin, so it's an important part of the process. You'll find it mainly in animal proteins (like milk and turkey) as well as in some other foods like bananas, nuts, seeds, oats, beans, and honey.

Calcium

This mineral plays a role in how our body utilizes tryptophan. It also helps regulate blood pressure and muscle movements, which are key to your being able to settle down when you get in bed. Dairy products are the best-known sources of calcium, but you'll also find it in dark leafy greens, tofu, and salmon. [61]

Vitamin B6
Vitamin B6 helps the body efficiently produce melatonin and serotonin, so it plays a big supporting role. Some good food sources are bananas, beans, fish, chicken, and whole grains.[62]

Carbohydrates
Carbohydrates are important for a few reasons. For starters, carbs enhance tryptophan levels in the blood. They're also important because a slight increase in insulin levels, which we experience when we eat carbs, actually helps the body fall asleep faster. Go for quality, though. Complex carbohydrates like beans, fruit, starchy vegetables like sweet potatoes, and whole grains will break down more slowly and keep your blood sugar stable so you don't wake up hungry in the middle of the night.

Potassium
This mineral soothes muscle aches and assists in the regulation of blood pressure and nerve function so you can fall asleep comfortably. Potassium is present in many foods, but some great ones to put on your list are avocados, bananas, tomatoes, oranges, and dark, leafy greens.[63]

Magnesium

Magnesium is a mineral that regulates blood pressure as well as muscle and nerve function and blood sugar. Magnesium is also thought to counteract the stress hormone cortisol, so it's a good one to pay attention to if stress in your brain and body make it hard for you to peacefully drift off at night. Some good food sources include bananas, nuts, spinach and other greens, chicken, fish, and dairy products.[64]

Easy Bedtime Snack Ideas

If you finish eating dinner within an hour or two of your bedtime, you may not need a bedtime snack, but if you find yourself needing a little something to help take the edge off, here are some great options to try.

A Banana

You might say that bananas are a bedtime superfood, thanks to their potassium, magnesium, vitamin B6, and tryptophan content. Add a teaspoon of your favorite nut butter for a little healthy fat.

Yogurt

Yogurt gives you a combination of calcium, magnesium, potassium, and tryptophan as well as some carbs (lactose) and protein. Just avoid flavored products, since sugar and artificial sweeteners can be hard on digestion. Sweeten with a teaspoon of honey instead for a little extra tryptophan.

A Hard-Boiled Egg

Eggs are an easy source of tryptophan as well as protein and fat. Also awesome: it's super easy to prep hard-boiled eggs ahead of time so you have them when you need them.

Cheese

Tina Fey's Liz Lemon in *30 Rock* was onto something with her "Night Cheese" routine. Cheese provides calcium and tryptophan, plus protein. To avoid going overboard, keep portions to about one ounce—that's about a quarter cup of soft cheese or an amount that's about the size of a tube of lipstick or a pair of dice for hard cheese. A fruit and cheese plate makes a lovely pre-bed snack.

Oats

Oatmeal might not sound like a bedtime snack, but it can actually be a great one. In addition to complex carbs, oats provide tryptophan and vitamin B6. An easy formula that will settle you down without being too filling is to cook a quarter cup of rolled or instant oats with a half cup of milk and some cinnamon for a bedtime snack. Add up to a teaspoon of honey if you need some sweetness, and if you need a little extra protein or fat to make it more filling, a teaspoon of your favorite nut butter.

Hummus with Veggies or Crackers

The chickpeas in hummus are a great plant-based source of tryptophan. This combo also provides carbohydrates and a little protein.

What to Avoid

Certain foods and beverages can also mess with your sleep.

Caffeine is a big one. Coffee, soda, energy drinks, and black and green tea are the most common sources, though some people who are very sensitive to caffeine may also find that chocolate impacts their sleep.

As we talked about in the chapter on finding your sweet spot with caffeine, setting a caffeine curfew for yourself—setting a time of day when you cut yourself off from caffeinated beverages—can make it possible for you to enjoy caffeine without risking it keeping you up at night. While some people might be able to have coffee at 4 p.m. and still get to bed without a problem, many people do better switching to decaf after 2 p.m., or even earlier.

Both eating a very large meal and attempting to go to bed when you're very hungry can make it hard to fall asleep. Some people may find that spicy foods, very sugary foods, and foods that are hard to digest (like high-fat meats, or fatty meals like a double-bacon cheeseburger and fries, or a rich dessert like a brownie sundae) also make falling asleep more difficult.

I'm not sure why the term "nightcap" is a thing because alcohol is another sleep saboteur. It would be awesome if a glass of wine or a stiff drink after a stressful day could help you sleep well, but, unfortunately, alcohol can actually disrupt your sleep.

Sure, you might fall asleep quickly, but have you noticed

how you tend to wake up in the middle of the night? That's because alcohol impacts the production of the different chemicals involved in our circadian rhythm, and it also blocks REM sleep, which is the restorative part of our sleep. Alcohol can also exacerbate breathing problems and lead to snoring, and may exacerbate sleep apnea. Then there's the fact that it's a diuretic, which means more bathroom trips in the middle of the night. Not exactly a recipe for a good night of rest.[65]

If you still want to enjoy an alcoholic drink, your best bet is to stick to a small amount and to enjoy it with a balanced meal, ideally where you have at least a few hours before you call it a night.

Other Things to Help You Get Better Sleep

Similarly to how exercise goes hand-in-hand with dietary changes when we're working toward a fitness goal, exercise can impact our sleep. I spoke with Dr. Sujay Kansagra, MD, an associate professor at Duke University Medical Center and director of the Duke Pediatric Neurology Sleep Medicine Program, about how sleep and exercise are linked. "Getting regular exercise can help you fall asleep faster and get better quality sleep. Exercise can also have beneficial effects on mood, anxiety, and stress, and these primary benefits can cause a secondary benefit to sleep as well," he told me. "But sleep can also impact exercise. Studies show that people tend to exercise less after a bad night of sleep."

When I asked whether the time of day you exercise

matters, he explained, "Most sleep doctors recommend trying to exercise earlier in the day if possible, and avoiding strenuous exercise close to bedtime. The reason is that exercise can cause an increase in the body's core temperature, and lowering your body temperature is good for helping you fall asleep. However, if your schedule is such that the only time in the day to exercise is in the evening, and you still find it easy to go to sleep, it's okay to go ahead and exercise."

While research has not uncovered any one magic type of exercise that's best for sleep, pay attention to any patterns related to how different activities impact your ability to drift off and stay asleep.

HYDRATE LIKE IT'S YOUR SIDE HUSTLE

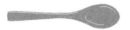

HYDRATION IS ABSOLUTELY vital to our health and well-being. I always tell my clients to hydrate like it's their side hustle. Your body requires adequate water to do all the work of taking care of you, from the nitty-gritty daily functioning of our cells we aren't even aware of, to effects we *can* see and feel, such as glowing skin and keeping your mind sharp. We also need water to regulate our body temperature, lubricate our joints, and protect our organs.

We often hear about water as something that can make us feel full and help us lose or maintain weight. That's because water takes up room in the stomach and, when it interacts with fiber, makes the fiber expand, which again takes up space. It's also important for digestion, as water helps keep everything moving smoothly through the digestive tract.

Thirst is often the first noticeable sign of dehydration. Other symptoms include foggy-headed or sluggish feelings, headaches, or irritability. Have you ever noticed how when you make the effort to drink some water when you feel that way, you perk up like a flower?

While there isn't an official recommendation for how much plain water you need,[66] there are some general guidelines about how much fluid you should consume—that includes what you get from foods and beverages.[67] Exactly how much depends on a lot of different factors like age and activity level as well as whether you have any underlying medical issues. For example, if you're very physically active, are sweating a lot, are experiencing vomiting or diarrhea, or have a fever, you'll need more.

There are a few different ways to calculate your individual needs, but a good jumping-off point for most healthy adults is to aim for 30-35 milliliters per kilogram (2.2 pounds) of body weight. To translate, for a 70 kilogram (154-pound) person, that's about 2100-2450 milliliters, or 70-82 ounces of fluid per day.

Too much math? To give yourself an easy starting place, take your weight in pounds, divide it by two, and that's your baseline in ounces. Tack on a little extra if you're very active or have anything else going on that could increase your needs. Divided into 8-ounce cups, 70 ounces is almost nine cups per day. If that sounds like a lot, remind yourself that fluids in foods (soup, fresh fruits and veggies, and so on) are included. Nonalcoholic and caffeine-free beverages also count toward your daily total.

Need to Up Your Water Intake?

If you need to increase your water intake, the right approach for you can depend on what your particular barrier is. Here are a few tips:

If You Hate the Taste of Water

Don't force it. Pretending to like plain water if you hate it sounds miserable. Instead, you can try to make it more interesting. A few things to try:

- add lemon, lime, or cucumber slices
- infuse it with fresh fruit or herbs
- try sparkling water

If You Just Can't Remember

Fitting hydration into things that are already part of your daily routine will make it automatic. For example, drink a glass of water when you're getting ready in the morning, have another with breakfast, and then a glass of water with each meal. You can work up to adding a glass between each meal if you need to.

If that just sounds like too much work, you could set alerts on your phone or place a note on your computer monitor, mirror, or another place you'll see a reminder to drink up.

If You're Too Busy

Convenience is key when you're super busy. Put a pitcher and a glass on your desk or keep a refillable bottle that's pleasing to look at in easy reach. If you're constantly on the go, invest in a refillable water bottle that will stay sealed and keep water at the temperature you prefer.

If remembering to refill said refillable container is the hard part for you, buy a liter of bottled water (or two, why not?) on your way to work and just make sure it's gone by the end of the day. To fill in the gaps, drink a glass before and after your workday.

SEE SUCCESS
BEYOND THE SCALE

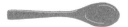

EVEN THOUGH WE know better, it's easy to fall into the trap of thinking that how much we weigh is the main measure of progress and success in our health journey. For that reason, it's not surprising that many people become overly fixated on the number on the scale.

Calling bullshit on this outdated idea is one of the first things I cover with my clients. While being at a healthy weight for your body is an appropriate goal, overall wellness is about so much more than your body mass index (BMI)—a body size measurement that takes into account your weight and height. Weight is just one component of a much larger picture—you also want to consider your energy and strength, as well as your mental and emotional state, how much stress and anxiety you feel, and how you handle it. Being above your ideal weight does not necessarily mean you're unhealthy, and it sure as hell doesn't mean you're not beautiful or worthy of love and happiness.

There is a lot of societal pressure to fit into very narrow beauty ideals. For example, there is a lot of pressure on women and female-identifying individuals to be as small as possible. For men, there's also a lot of emphasis placed on being in shape and to have very low body fat relative to muscle mass. Eating disorders among men have been on the rise in recent years. However, weight loss doesn't have to be a part of a healthy living plan. For example, even if you eventually want to lose a few pounds but are struggling with stress eating, maybe your priority is to get a handle on what's stressing you out first before you feel ready to start thinking about weight. Or maybe you're comfortable at your weight but want to have more energy and start making food choices that support that goal.

Just as an FYI, though, if you're tracking your weight as part of your health plan, the best time to do it is first thing in the morning, right after you've used the bathroom, and without any clothes on. This will give you the most accurate number. It's also a good idea to use the same scale every time, as there can be discrepancies from one to the other. That's also why weighing yourself on vacation won't really tell you much.

Here are a few tips that have helped my clients dial down the drama around the numbers on the scale.

Inches

If numbers are helpful, consider tracking changes in your measurements rather than simply your weight. This can be really easy if you're incorporating exercise into your routine. Because muscle weighs more than fat, it's not uncommon to see the number on the scale stay the same or even go up as you build more muscle, even if you're seeing changes in your body composition and losing inches from your midsection, hips, thighs, and so on.

Depending on the types of exercise you do, you may notice that certain areas like your arms get bigger and more defined, but if you're someone who gets upset by higher numbers, skip that one. This is a good thing to measure at longer intervals, such as monthly or quarterly.

Body Fat Percentage

Speaking of body composition, a great measure of progress is changes in your body fat percentage. You might have memories of a little pincher caliper thing your Phys. Ed. teacher demo-ed in gym class back in the day, but now you can easily purchase a digital scale that measures body composition. This is another good one to track monthly or quarterly, especially if your goal is to decrease your body fat as you build lean muscle.

A Piece of Clothing

Pretty much everyone has an item of clothing in their closet that feels like an accurate measure of where they're at with their weight and fitness goals—I like to call them "honesty pants" (you know the pair I'm talking about), but you could also use a shirt, a dress, or something else. Someone on a weight-loss journey might choose to hang on to an item of clothing in the largest size they own and occasionally try it on to remind themselves of how far they've come. You can use this method as frequently or infrequently as feels helpful to you, but note that you'll notice more pronounced changes when you have longer intervals.

Fitness Progress

Some people can find it incredibly motivating to note changes in things like the amount of weight they can lift, the number of miles they can comfortably walk, or the amount of time they can shave off their usual run. An app or journal can be a useful tool to help you track progress over time.

Your Energy Levels

It's important to pay attention to changes in your energy level. Pick a specific time (or times) of day and, using a 1-10 scale, check in with yourself. While you could do this daily, you could also do it weekly or monthly if preferred. Again, you can track your results using a journal or an app. However you do it, chances are, over time, you'll notice some patterns.

Your Connection to Your Body

This is a big one for people who struggle with things like compulsive or mindless eating, or who have a tendency to numb out and lose connection with how they're feeling in their body during times of stress. Noting how in touch you are with things like your hunger and fullness cues, your perception of pain (something we may tune out when we're in that fight-or-flight mode), and your awareness of how your body responds to different activities can tell you a lot about how far you've come in learning how to shift your own energy. A few ways to work this into your routine: Mindfulness practices like meditation, things like putting your fork down between bites, or doing check-ins with yourself at regular intervals to see what sensations you're feeling and what they're telling you.

Your Stress and Anxiety Levels

Similar to our energy levels, our perception of how stressed or anxious we feel can tell us so much about our progress and clue us in to what sets us off and why. A scale or other method of documenting your stress levels can be helpful in tracking progress over time. That said, if there are certain situations you know you struggle with, those can be a good benchmark. For me, technology issues have, at times, sent me into a tailspin—I know I'm in a good place when something goes wrong and I can just calmly deal with it rather than have a meltdown.

MAKE EXERCISE PART OF YOUR STRESS-MANAGEMENT ROUTINE

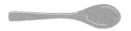

EXERCISE IS ONE of the most effective tools in your stress management toolbox.[68] Unfortunately, it often falls by the wayside when we're overwhelmed or wigged out.

If you've ever fallen into that mind-set of "I'm too busy putting out fires at work to make time," or you feel pressured to tend to everyone else's needs, or you feel guilty when you sneak away for a few minutes, or you tell yourself the story that you'll get back into a routine when a particular situation calms down, you've likely experienced how much worse you feel physically (and possibly also mentally and emotionally). Getting back to being physically active can also feel much more daunting after you've taken time away. Other common deterrents include lack of confidence or worrying about what others will think of your performance.

How Exercise Can Help You Manage Stress

The research is absolutely conclusive, though, that making exercise a regular part of your routine has multiple benefits to the brain and body. Here are a few examples:

Endorphins Boost Your Mood

Endorphins are feel-good neurotransmitters that are released during physical activity—the "high" in the "runner's high," if you will, though you don't have to choose running as your go-to activity. Almost any form of movement can cause a release of endorphins, which will make you feel instantly happier. Endorphins are also known to interact with receptors in the brain that reduce our perception of pain. They also act as sedatives, helping us calm down if we're stressed or feeling anxious.

Exercise May Help Improve Self-Esteem

Being regularly active and sticking to a routine you enjoy can increase your confidence and feeling of well-being. The sense of accomplishment can spill over into other areas of your life. For people who enjoy group fitness classes, that sense of community or camaraderie can also be a connector that's important for self-esteem.

Exercise Can Serve as a Form of Meditation

Have you ever noticed how much clearer your head feels after a walk? Do you find that you get a lot of creative ideas while you're working out, or suddenly have the mental bandwidth to come up with a solution to an issue that's been plaguing you? These are a few examples of the meditative effect of movement—by helping you get out of your head and into your body, decluttering the mind.

You May Sleep Better

Regular moderate physical activity has also been shown to improve sleep, which is key to having energy and feeling like you can withstand challenges in life. Because sleep deprivation has been associated with increased risk of physical and mental health issues, making exercise a part of your healthy sleep protocol may also improve your overall wellness.

Which Type of Exercise Is Best?

We'll get more into this in another chapter, but the short answer is that any form of physical activity you enjoy and that helps you feel strong, energized, and happy deserves a regular place in your routine.

There's a lot of information out there about which types of exercise are best for helping you achieve specific goals, but especially if you're just starting to establish a workable routine, focus on what you enjoy the most and can realistically fit into your life. So often, I've seen clients try to implement a regimen they found online or that was recommended by a friend, only to wind up giving it up because they didn't really enjoy it, found it hard to make time, or felt like it just didn't fit into their daily routine.

A 2008 poll by the American Psychological Association showed that the preferred forms of exercise for stress management were walking, running, and yoga[69] but anything that works for you can be an effective part of your stress management plan.

Be Open to Needing Other Tools

Hiring a trainer or joining a group or class that you enjoy can offer the education, accountability, and support you need to get into a consistent exercise routine. We'll get more into this in another chapter, but there are tons of options at all kinds of price points and to fit all different schedules. You can dip your toes or dive right in—up to you.

All that said, if you find yourself struggling with serious depression or anxiety that interferes with your daily functioning, seek help from a mental health professional. While exercise may be an effective tool, you may require additional forms of treatment such as talk therapy or meditation to produce the results you need.

TURN YOUR OWN DIAL: HOW TO TAP INTO YOUR MOTIVATION

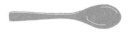

OKAY, SO YOU'VE heard all about how awesome exercise is and how important self-care is, but what if you lack the time, energy, or motivation to lace up your sneakers, do a healthy food prep, book a spa appointment, or schedule dinner with an inspiring friend?

As we talked about in the chapter on the power of intention, reframing self-care as a tool in your toolbox as opposed to treating it like a task you need to cross off a list can go a long way toward making it part of your routine. It's not all salt baths and yoga retreats, either—self-care can be as basic as taking thirty minutes to prep some food for the week or asking a friend if they want to do a workout class together instead of grabbing drinks (or you could always do barre and *then* the bar . . .).

Tapping into the motivation to take care of yourself goes beyond wanting to look a certain way physically or hitting an arbitrary milestone. Treating self-care as a non-negotiable and rewarding yourself for fitting it into your regular week as opposed to looking at it as a special treat or something you can do only after other tasks is also key. When you can really see the deeper value in how nurturing your mental, physical, and spiritual well-being can help you be more resilient and have a better experience in your personal and professional life, it becomes much easier to make it a priority.

I spoke with Kindbody president Annbeth Eschbach, who is also the founder of Exhale Spa, about the value of empowering yourself to shift your own energy and turn the dial back in a positive direction when you need to. "I'm a big believer in how important and vital energy is to being a flourishing human being," she says. "Let's face it, we all go through really tough ups and downs all of the time, and recognizing that and figuring out how to turn your own dial to influence yourself is such a game changer in life."

Want to learn how? Here are some tips to get you started.

Tune into What Shifts Your Energy

The list of things that shift our energy is as individual as we are. To share a personal example, I know I'm really sensitive to music, so if I'm having a hard day or feeling low, I've learned to turn on some tunes that make me feel good and to save the Elliott Smith and Leonard Cohen for another time.

When you can feel yourself getting swept off track, says Eschbach, acknowledge and understand what's happening, and turn to those things that you've learned shift your energy back in a positive direction.

"For most human beings, the levers are fairly simple: It's moving, it's connecting, it's being touched, it's lying down and relaxing and taking some deep breaths, it's sweating something out, and then feeling a sense of accomplishment."

What things give you that sense of accomplishment? If it's helpful, make a list. You can also note which ones are free and which ones cost money—and how much. This list can serve as a building block for your own self-care budget, so to speak.

Remember: You Have a Choice

While you might get overwhelmed, Eschbach acknowledges, you can control how you respond to what's going on around you and what energy you give out. "You have a choice—you can either be magnetic and compelling or you can be angry and toxic and stressed out. In my past, I really got caught up in thinking stress was cool and allowing that to fuel me." It was learning about our ability to rewire the brain through moments of mindfulness and gratitude and smiling and being touched, she explains, that finally enabled her to feel a shift in herself.

She adds that she believes that "People who are able to be present and listen to other people and smile and be grateful are so much more effective because of it than people who are so anxious to prove themselves and compete and stand out."

Start Small

In her previous job before founding Exhale, Eschbach says

she was traveling every single week, and she noticed she would work herself into a negative mind-set from the second she got into yet another cab to go to yet another airport. "I had these mental conversations with myself that got me tied up in knots."

Finally, one day, she decided to try an experiment, "I said, 'I'm going to go to the airport and I'm going to smile from the minute I walk in to the moment I get on that airplane.'" She was so struck by how positively everyone around her responded and by what a positive experience she had, that she knew she couldn't go back to her old pattern.

"I needed to figure out how to flourish in everyday accessible ways that happened in small snippets. So I started playing with it. I would feel the physiological change that would come over me from behaving differently. It was pretty powerful." That shift—and Eschbach's experience of tapping into her ability to make it happen for herself—became the inspiration for Exhale.

So often, I hear my clients, friends, and family complain about not having enough time to work out or cook, for example, but when we dig into it a little more, it becomes clear that they're caught up in thinking they need to spend a lot of time on those things.

I love introducing them to workable solutions like meal and grocery delivery services and online or app-based workouts they can do from virtually anywhere with minimal, if any, equipment. We come up with lists of healthy takeout options and highlight inconsistencies in the stories we tell ourselves.

One of my favorites is that, in the same five minutes you spend ordering unhealthy takeout, you can order something else that better supports your goals. Or how is it that you have ten minutes to spend scrolling on social media (which, let's be real, often makes you feel like crap) but "can't" make time for a ten-minute stretch or quick strength workout?

"The world is changing," says Eschbach. "There's so much out there that allows you to do this in more accessible, smaller bites." You're also seeing more wellness and fitness businesses start to cater more to the needs of people with less time by offering shorter classes and services and products designed to be more portable.

Use Positive Reinforcement

You don't have to be that person bragging about their run on social media if that stuff makes you roll your eyes, but allowing yourself to enjoy a sense of accomplishment can help you stay motivated on those days when you don't want to get out of bed or fire up the stove after a long day at work.

Having people in your life to cheer you on and remind you to take care of yourself can also be incredibly valuable. Even an alert on your phone to give you a boost of encouragement or ask if you're staying hydrated can help.

"The more we get reminders from one another or from our own communities and families or even from our phones, the more this is going to be integrated into the fabric of everyone's lives. I think we will have a much more well world," says Eschbach. This desire to build in a "rewards" system was a main reason Exhale partnered with World of Hyatt to offer a program where participants could use points for their travel and their wellness needs.

It might feel weird at first, but practice telling yourself how proud you are of yourself and how great you feel for taking time out of your day to take care of yourself. Chances are, not only do you benefit from that, but so do the others in your life.

Make It a Group Thing

Live and interactive digital group experiences in fitness, meditation, and wellness have become very popular even as isolation becomes more of a public health issue. Eschbach explains, "People are far more drawn to these communal and social experiences than ever before because we're so, you know, whacked out on technology. Everybody is so lonely."

As someone who works alone most of the time and has lived alone on and off for so much of my adult life, community is key. Sure, I go to favorite fitness studios for the classes, but it was really about connecting with other people there and building relationships. Learning to meditate in a group setting made it so much more approachable than just sitting by myself, staring into a candle, wondering if I was doing it right. Taking a walk with a friend or colleague is also a favorite way to connect and fit movement into my day.

If you struggle with getting motivated to work out or cook on your own, find a class or pair up with a pal. Making it a shared experience might just be the change you need.

FIND YOUR GO-TO PRE- AND POST-WORKOUT SNACKS

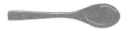

WHEN IT COMES to enjoying a healthy life and meeting your fitness and wellness goals, diet and exercise go hand in hand. Knowing what to eat before and after your workouts can give you the energy you need to get the most out of your time and support post-exercise recovery so you can reap the benefits of your efforts.

To be very general, it comes down to having an optimal balance of protein and carbs. The ratio varies a bit depending on the type of physical activity and how soon before or after you're eating, but once you get into a good routine, you'll find that it's pretty intuitive. You also want to pay attention to hydration and make sure to replenish lost electrolytes (electrically charged minerals and compounds that are essential for normal body functions—a few common ones are sodium, chloride, potassium, and magnesium) if you're doing intense activity, but the good news is that for your everyday workouts, you don't need to buy lots of expensive products—in most cases, everyday foods will cover your bases just fine. Bottom line: The better you feel, the more motivated you'll be to keep a good thing going, and the proper fuel can help.

What to Eat Before a Workout

Not being adequately fueled could cause you to lose steam earlier or keep you from performing at your peak potential. This is absolutely key if you're doing something intense like cardio (think: running, swimming, or cycling), strength training, or something like martial arts, dance, or a class where there are many repetitive movements and you'll be exerting a lot of energy.

While you can often get away with skipping a snack if you're doing a lower-intensity activity first thing in the morning or within a couple hours of your last meal, you're still going to get the most energy bang for your buck if you eat a little something beforehand. And don't forget to hydrate, especially if you're going to be sweating a lot.

Carbs are the star of the pre-workout show, because our bodies need the glucose they provide for energy. As a general rule, you want to eat easily digestible carbohydrates before a workout. Be careful with high-fiber, high-protein, and high-fat foods if you're eating less than an hour before your workout, since they can cause GI discomfort. If you've got an hour or more before your workout, protein will give you some staying power.

Many fitness and health care professionals break it down into grams of carbohydrate and protein. Here's a formula that can be a helpful guide:

- *Thirty minutes before*: 15-30 grams of carbohydrate, minimal protein; or a 3:1 carbs to protein ratio (so if your snack has up to 5 grams of protein, then aim for 15 grams of carbs). You don't need to overload protein—it's been shown that the body can't absorb more than about 20-30 grams in one meal.
- *One hour before*: 30-70 grams of carbohydrates, or a 2:1 carbs to protein ratio
- *Two hours before*: Have a normal, balanced meal

That said, your needs may vary, so if you find that you're having trouble finding your sweet spot, check in with a sports dietitian or a trainer who's certified in sports nutrition.

What It Looks Like in Real Life
Here are a few examples of pre-workout foods to try. In each category, any one of the bulleted examples would cover your nutritional needs.

Thirty minutes before:

- A large banana or two small pieces of fruit
- A slice of toast with one tablespoon of jam or hummus
- A quarter cup of dried fruit
- Half a nut-and-fruit-based bar

Sixty minutes before:

- A PB&J sandwich
- A piece of fruit with a tablespoon of nut butter
- Two pieces of toast and a cooked egg
- One cup of a low-fiber cereal with 1 cup of milk or three-quarters cup of plain yogurt
- Half a cup of cooked oatmeal made with milk or topped with a tablespoon of nut butter
- A quarter cup of trail mix made with nuts and dried fruit or a nut-and-fruit bar
- One medium sweet potato topped with 1 tablespoon of nut butter

All that said, if you have a go-to pre-workout snack that doesn't fit those guidelines, what matters most is that it works for you and helps you meet your goals.

What to Eat After a Workout

After a workout, protein is super important. It helps provide the amino acids your body needs to repair and rebuild. You still need carbs, though, to help replenish the body's glycogen stores (glycogen is a complex carbohydrate comprised of several glucose molecules). Just be sure to choose ones that will provide lots of nutrients, such as minimally processed whole grains, beans, and other complex carbs like starchy veggies (sweet potato, corn) and fruit.

Milk is actually another source of carbohydrates, thanks to the lactose in there.

If you're feeling super hungry after a tough workout, be mindful of how you refuel. You just put in a lot of hard work, so show your body some love with foods that will nourish it. You might have burned a lot of calories, but when replenishing them, your body will definitely notice the difference between, say, 200 calories of a well-balanced snack and 200 calories from a sugary coffee drink.

You don't have to make yourself crazy over timing and grams of protein and carbs, but aim for a mix of the two, and ideally, eat something within an hour after completing your workout. What's most important, though, is to refuel before you hit that point where you're, like, "I'm so hungry and wiped out I'm just going to curl up here on the floor and cry." You also don't need to be chugging giant recovery smoothies or eating expensive protein bars after a workout.

Prioritize what makes you feel satisfied and fits into the context of your day. For example, if you work out in the morning but it makes more sense for you to have breakfast at your desk, have a small post-workout snack like protein powder shaken up with water or even a latte or cappuccino, which provides both carbs and protein if you have it made with cow's milk. Have Breakfast Part 2 later in the morning, when it's more convenient. Again, I really do believe that the body is smart and lets us know what feels good, but generally speaking, a good meal to eat after your average workout would include protein, some fiber-rich complex carbohy-drates, and healthy fats.

If numbers are helpful, aim for a 3:1 or a 2:1 ratio of carbs to protein. For example, a peanut butter sandwich would give you roughly 30 grams of carbs and 10 grams of protein.

Snack Ideas:

- A piece of fruit and a hard-boiled egg or piece of cheese
- A slice of toast with peanut butter or an egg
- 8 ounces milk
- Whole grain cereal with milk
- 6 ounces of plain yogurt with half a banana or half a cup of berries

Meal Ideas:

- A veggie omelet and whole wheat toast or half a cup of roasted sweet potato
- Oatmeal with ground flax, fruit, and 2 tablespoons of nuts or 1 tablespoon of nut butter
- A small whole wheat wrap with egg or egg whites and veggies
- Plain Greek yogurt with fruit and honey and almond slivers
- A smoothie with fruit and milk (add protein powder

if you're using a low-protein plant-based milk like almond or coconut)

- Half a cup of beans, brown rice, quinoa, or other whole grains or starchy vegetables with green veggies and a serving of meat, fish, or an egg, plus a quarter of an avocado or a tablespoon of tahini for healthy fat
- A sandwich made with whole wheat bread and lean protein such as turkey, ham, or chicken

Over time, you'll find the options that'll work for you. Listen to your body. It does so much to take care of you, so return the favor.

HOW TO MAKE TIME FOR FITNESS IN YOUR DAY

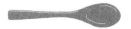

RAISE YOUR HAND if you've ever felt like you had no time to exercise. What about if you've ever felt guilty about taking time away from something "more important" to move your body?

We've already talked about the benefits of exercise, but let's dig a little deeper into how to actually make time and space in a schedule that feels relentlessly full. Here are a few easy ways to do just that.

Put It in Your Calendar
Pre-booking classes that have a cancellation fee or making plans with a friend are just a few ways to reduce the chance that you'll change your mind and back out.

Break Workouts into Smaller Blocks of Time
The Department of Health and Human Services recommends aiming for at least 150 minutes of moderate aerobic activity or 75 minutes of vigorous aerobic activity per week—or a combination of moderate and vigorous, so

you can spread that out in a way that works for your life-style.

Exercise does not have to take an hour. Take the pressure off and give yourself permission to work in shorter bursts of activity, say by doing five or ten minutes at a time through your day, if that's what you can manage.

Choose Workouts You Actually Enjoy

It's harder to make time for something you loathe, so choose activities you enjoy.

Make It Easy

Having the clothes and gear you need ready to go cuts down on time spent gathering your stuff together. Lay out your workout clothes the night before a morning workout or keep your gym bag in your car so you can get there on your lunch break or right after work.

Reward Yourself

As we talked about in the chapter on shifting your own energy, using positive reinforcement, cheering yourself on, and rewarding yourself for working out can encourage you to make it a habit.

THE BEST WORKOUT IS THE ONE YOU'LL ACTUALLY DO

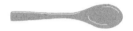

AS IT IS with many things in life, it's not about having time, it's about making time for exercise. Have you ever noticed that even when your life feels insane, you somehow manage to fit in the people and activities you care about?

Or maybe you've been in a situation where someone you're interested in keeps saying they've "been so busy with work/school/family" until you finally get the hint that, actually, they just don't want to see you anymore.

It's the same thing when it comes to physical activity. You're much more likely to make it happen when the type of exercise is something you genuinely want to do.

That said, give yourself a variety of options. Too often, I see people getting bored or burned out doing the same thing over and over, or becoming so set in their routine that they can't cope when they have to be flexible. Having a few different types of activity in your life that you enjoy can help you feel more well-rounded. There are also certain workouts that are best for different moods and energy levels.

While exercise is an important part of my own self-care

routine, I'm not a certified expert, so I spoke to a few people who are, like Johari Mayfield, a certified personal trainer who has a dance background and works with adults and children, and Lauren Chiarello Mika, founder of Chi Chi Life, fitness instructor and a two-time cancer survivor, who is also a fundraising and events guru and marathoner.

Here are some of their tips for finding (or discovering) what you love.

Aim for Whole Body Fitness

Neither Chiarello nor Mayfield believes that there is one "best" workout—"I don't want to 'yuck anyone's yum,'" says Mayfield. But having a combination of cardiovascular activity and strengthening (whether in one exercise session or spread throughout the week) helps support overall wellness. "Cardio helps you build up heart strength and cardiovascular capability while strength training helps build bone density, core strength, as well as flexibility and mobility through joints and muscles," explains Chiarello.

While it's easy to buy into the hype that exercise is about looking hot, being active also helps prepare us for the movements we do in our day-to-day life so we avoid injury. Mayfield often works "movements that are compound, multi-joint actions (like a push-up, pull-up, deadlift, or squat)" into her sessions, along with those that "require you to change the level of your body, such as bending down to the floor and moving through different planes." She adds, "I had a physical therapist tell me once to watch and really observe children and how they move around a playground. That's how we should be moving during our workout. They don't move linearly. Curves, bends, these are all movements that happen throughout the day. There's something to be said about looking good, she says, but it's also about not being in a surgeon's office.

Keep an Open Mind

We often tell ourselves stories about what we do and don't do, sometimes without having given what's on the "no" list a real shot. You might even be pleasantly surprised by what you like. "Try it all and find what energizes you," says Chiarello. Of course, you don't have to love everything. "I love to try new things, and then I assess whether it felt like it was for me and if I would go back." She adds that if you're taking a class, try a few different instructors and see whether a different teaching style resonates more with you than others.

Another thing to keep in mind is that your interests and preferences may shift over time. Sometimes I see people tie up their identity and self-worth in their chosen sport or activity, and in the unfortunate event of an injury or illness (or if they stop loving that activity), it can be incredibly difficult, emotionally, to accept that they're taking a break or are ready to move on. Give yourself permission to go with the ebbs and flows and to follow your instincts about what feels good and what doesn't.

To give you a personal example, in my twenties, I did a

ton of cardio and hot yoga. An arm injury when I was twenty-four led me to a physical therapist who recommended Pilates to help me build core strength and avoid future injuries. I never would have tried it otherwise, but I fell in love. Experiencing burnout and a back injury a few years later was what finally got me to dial down the cardio and get even more intentional about strength training and flexibility as key parts of my regular routine.

If you're intimidated by the prospect of going to a group class, Chiarello recommends inviting a friend or, if you're going solo, to be patient with yourself and be encouraging instead of fixating on feeling like you're not doing well. "One of the biggest pieces of my teaching is making people feel welcome and applauding them for trying something new. It takes a lot of grit to show up!"

Think Positively

Approaching exercise with a positive attitude and being patient with yourself can help you have a much better experience. Chiarello explains, "We can really psych ourselves out, but if we come from a place of acceptance and arriving as we are, we do the best we can. When we decide and choose that's enough and continue to show up consistently, that's when change will happen." She also is a believer in the power of community as a source of positive energy and inspiration.

Mayfield, who also teaches group classes, wants students to feel welcome. "I just want people to feel comfortable in their body and personal space and within their community. Anybody who may feel they don't measure up, yes you do! Movement belongs to everybody."

She cautions her clients to be careful when scrolling through social media for inspiration. "Photoshop is real! ... Stop following social media accounts that make you feel bad when you look at them." She adds, "As often as possible, be with real people when you exercise so you can see how the body works. Real time and online time are two different things. In real life, things are not rehearsed, lit, and in costume."

Mix It Up Depending on Your Mood

Our mood can also impact our workout experience—and vice versa. Movement can shift our energy in the direction we need it to. "I think it depends on the person," says Chiarello, but it's worth trying out different workouts to see what you respond to. "If one person is feeling stressed, they may feel they need to go get a run in, but someone else might want to go to yoga to help them feel more grounded and connected to their breath." She recommends experimenting with various forms of exercise and journaling pre- and postworkout to help you tune into what really works for you—and to unload your thoughts and feelings so you can work through them.

Mayfield agrees that both calming and more vigorous forms of exercise have their place. "For me, yoga helps to calm my central nervous system down. When I'm feeling afraid or anxious, I like to do yoga so I learn how to breathe through things. It helps me put a pause or slow down my response to something that might make me feel angry or anxious."

"In terms of channeling other aggressions like anger in a way that's more dynamic," she recommends cardio, boxing, and drumming while dancing. The drumming, in particular, offers the added benefit of creating sound, which can also be therapeutic. With drumming, she says, "You're doing something that's getting the energy out but that's also artistic, and you're connecting with others and creating sound."

When you're feeling fired-up or pissed off, a high-intensity class like spinning, kickboxing, or a weights class could help you deal. Mayfield explains, "Where aggression is an emotion that's expected in a class, it's healthy to get it out through movement."

When you feel like your brain is on overload, a slower or low-impact workout like a yoga flow or Pilates class may be a good fit. A walk around the block can also be great if you just feel like you need to clear your head to cool off after an argument or annoying email.

How to Deal When You're Lacking Motivation

Even the most committed exercise enthusiasts have days when motivating themselves is harder than others. Chiarello encourages, "Move through excuses, show up, do what you can, and know that it's better than nothing." If you're feeling discouraged because you're still in the early stages of working toward a fitness goal, give yourself some grace. "When we come from a place of acceptance and arriving as we are, good things will come. Change doesn't happen overnight, and in this landscape we're living in now, people want things quickly, but change takes time. You need to put in the work to see results, like any other area of your life. Progress takes time. You have to put in the time, energy, and dedication in order to flourish."

Making plans with a friend also adds a level of accountability and support. "That person is depending on you, and you're depending on each other," she says. "A sense of camaraderie is built. I would recommend trying to find a community. Maybe that scares some people, but there are a lot of great communities. That could even be on social media if not in person, where you share the exercises you're doing that week."

If you're struggling to get moving, Mayfield also recommends calling a friend. "It gets us out of ourselves. At a certain point, self-will will fail, and then once that self-will starts to wane a bit more, you have that second thing of, 'Well, I gave my word to my friend that we were going to do this thing,' that provides another kind of motivation." Yes, it's about being motivated to stay on point with your own goals, she explains, but it also becomes about helping someone to move forward with theirs as well.

Mayfield also recommends hiring a personal trainer to provide that financial incentive or joining classes to stay motivated. It provides a sense of community, she says. "You know you're going to see your friends, you'll more than likely get dressed for the occasion, so there's other kinds of emotional payback you get on top of the workout."

Don't Feel Like You Have to Spend a Ton of Time or Money

"There's this phrase people use about 'making time,'" says Chiarello. "If only we could literally make it. We'd be millionaires. I prefer to say 'carve out time,' and dedicating that time you're able to spend. Life will ebb and flow. Do what you can. You've got to make exercise a priority and move through the excuses. It's a matter of showing up for yourself so you can show up for others."

"We all have twenty-four hours in a day," she explains, "and we choose how we spend those." It can feel like our time for ourselves can be extremely limited, but carving out thirty minutes (or less, if that's all you have) is well worth it. "I promise you will feel better and stronger. If you're putting yourself first, all your other relationships will benefit. When you carve out that time for yourself, you're able to be more present in your day to day activities."

Don't have thirty minutes? Chiarello says, "Even fifteen minutes or doing a plank by your bedside in your pajamas for one minute counts. I love planks!"

To make exercise more financially accessible, she's also a fan of low-cost electronic sources like interactive programs, accountability groups, and streaming workout videos. Scoping out free events in your community can also be a great way to connect with others while enjoying exercise.

Mayfield is also a fan of online resources if you just don't have the time or wherewithal to leave the house. She also encourages people to start with "real easy tasks, one task at a time. Then build from there." Even doing laundry or using household items as weights can work. "The kitchen is so full of opportunities. I have a client using a wine bottle, a bottle of bleach—you don't have to have the traditional weights to get the strength training in there. Use commercial breaks as a time to get in squats, jumping jacks, lunges, plank-jacks, crunches. Keep it simple."

FIND A SUNSCREEN YOU LOVE

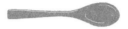

WHEN I WAS doing my neurology rotation as an intern in the hospital, I had a patient I'll never forget. They were a young person about my age whose malignant melanoma had metastasized to her brain. It's been so many years since, but I can still remember the family members' faces and the little details they shared with me about how healthy the patient had been in all other areas of her life before getting skin cancer.

That same summer, I had a precancerous mole excised from my chest. You learn the difference between getting something cut *off* and getting something cut *out* when it involves sutures. I was doing my cardiac rotation by then, so walking into patients' rooms with a big mess of gauze and tape over my own heart (a lab coat can only hide so much) made for quite the icebreaker.

While I never used a tanning bed or intentionally tried to tan growing up, I definitely got a little bit lax about applying and reapplying sunscreen. Sure, you could say genetics play a role (I'm super pale and, like my dad was, prone to growing all manner of suspicious moles), but being mindful about sun exposure and regularly applying sunscreen are your best defenses.

If you've ever had to have a mole biopsied or removed, you know how the stress and anxiety swirl around in your brain. In the weeks waiting for test results, I lost a lot of sleep worrying about just how bad the situation was. The recovery time after the procedure was brutal too. I hadn't thought to ask about what to expect and whether I would need pain medication, and I was so sore and bruised. Even the smallest movement was excruciating. I also kept having to go back because the supposedly dissolvable sutures kept popping out to the surface of the skin and needed to get plucked away.

Why am I telling you this? I could probably have saved myself so much worrying and pain if I had just worn my freaking sunscreen. I still have a big scar on my chest that serves as a daily reminder to apply it.

I have the sunscreen conversation with pretty much all of my clients at some point. Protecting your skin from the sun is one of the most important things you can do for your health, and it takes almost zero time. Aside from protecting you from cancer, it can also help you avoid wrinkles, hyperpigmentation, and all that stuff you don't think about until it's too late. And for anybody who wants to argue that we get vitamin D from the sun, I would say that we can still get what we need from food and supplements. Yes, sunlight allows us to synthesize vitamin D, but at what cost?

One of the biggest barriers to wearing sunscreen as a regular part of your self-care routine, though, is hating the way it feels, looks, or smells. The goal is to find something you can wear comfortably and even enjoy applying every day. What works for one person may not be the magic fit for someone else, and that's okay.

To help make it easier to solve that problem, I spoke with Mandi Nyambi, the author of *Fresh Face* and cofounder of Baalm, a service that matches users with their dream skincare products through skin testing and preference tracking.

Take the Time to Get to Know Your Skin

We spend so much time focused on getting our skin to behave the way it's "supposed to" according to societal standards that prize a perfectly smooth, even-toned complexion, Nyambi explains. Part of her company's mission is to help women "understand the science of what our skin is trying to tell us, as opposed to trying to attack" those things we don't like. "There's nothing 'wrong' with a pimple or hyperpigmentation, but there is something wrong with ignoring what your skin is trying to tell you." Is your skin sensitive? Acne-prone? Oily? Combination? Does it change with the seasons or—a common one for women—throughout your menstrual cycle? These are just a few of the things to become familiar with.

Identifying which products you like and which ones your skin reacts poorly to will also give you valuable information about the ingredients and qualities to look for in a sunscreen. "When you find products that do work, compare ingredient labels and see if there are similar ingredients in there," says Nyambi. "Even if it's just starting with the first ten ingredients in the bottle and trying to understand, it will go a long way" in helping you find your match.

She adds, "Using labels like acne-prone, oily, and dry skin can help, but don't be afraid to dip into the other categories. Just because it's not marketed to you doesn't mean it won't work for you."

Choose Your Class

There are two main classes of sunscreen, Nyambi explains: physical and chemical. "Physical sunscreens work to reflect and scatter UV radiation," she says, "and chemical sunscreen absorbs it and then releases it as heat off your body."

Physical sunscreen contains active mineral ingredients such as zinc oxide and/or titanium dioxide (both of which are naturally broad spectrum) and because it works by sitting on the skin and deflecting radiation, it starts to work as soon as you apply it.

Chemical sunscreens, because they have to penetrate the skin before they can start working, take about 20 minutes to sink in after you apply. Some people may find these more irritating than physical sunscreens, as different ingredients have to be combined in order to achieve that full spectrum coverage.

Physical sunscreens have been gaining in popularity

over recent years as research has continued to highlight the benefits of physical sunscreen and product innovation has led to more approachable options. Nyambi explains, "Physical sunscreen may be good for people with sensitive skin, acne, or rosacea. They also tend to be a bit more mattifying," so if you don't like chemical sunscreens or how they make your skin look, it's a good alternative.

Choose the Right SPF—and Apply Smartly

SPF stands for "sun protection factor," which measures how long the sun will protect you from ultraviolet B rays, which cause skin reddening, sunburn, and skin damage and can contribute to skin cancer. You can find SPF levels ranging from 4 to 100 (probably higher), but Nyambi says that research has shown 30-50 is the most effective. "Anything above that is unnecessary, but you do need to reapply."

How much you need isn't always clear, but health experts recommend that to cover your entire face and body, the amount that would fill a shot glass is a good guideline. Don't forget areas like your hairline, scalp, behind the ears, your nose, lips, hands, the back of your ears and neck, and the tops of your feet.[70]

One area where there has been a lot of innovation, Nyambi says, is in applicator types. The most common ones you'll see are still the creams, sticks, and sprays, but there are other options now like brushes and compacts. Nyambi is also excited about new products like clear sunscreen and gels.

233

Other Sun Protection FYIs

Apply sunscreen thirty minutes before sun exposure and reapply at least every two hours—more frequently if you've been sweating a lot or swimming. Waterproof sunscreens are also available.

Making your sun protection routine as convenient and enjoyable as possible to stick to is well worth the effort. Finding your dream sunscreen is an important step, but you'll need to invest in a few other essentials as well, such as a wide-brimmed hat. Train yourself to be smart about when you go in the sun and when you reapply sunscreen. If you need to, setting an alert on your phone or asking a friend to remind you—whatever works—can help keep you covered.

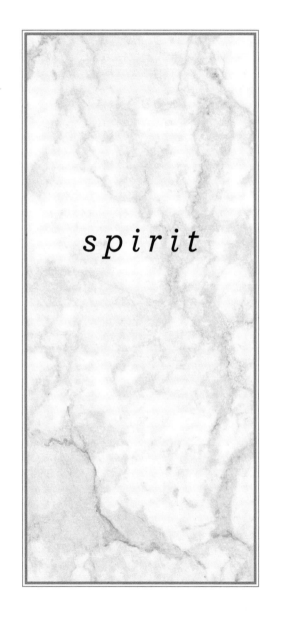

spirit

HAVE A LONELINESS
GAME PLAN

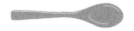

EVERYBODY GETS LONELY sometimes. Whether you're an introvert, extrovert, married, single, old, or young—it's just one of those annoyingly inevitable parts of life. Aside from the fact that feeling blue is unpleasant, it can also trigger some unhelpful coping mechanisms that can tear down our self-esteem and undermine any progress we've made toward our health and wellness goals. Eating to combat loneliness—especially eating unhealthy "comfort foods"—is very common; so is drinking. Some other examples of when a comforting activity can become a problem: binge-watching TV, playing video games, or gambling to the point where other things in your life slide.

As I wrote about earlier in the book, shopping is one I know *I* have to be careful not to turn to when I'm feeling lonely. That's why when my clients talk about raiding the vending machine or hitting up the candy aisle at the drugstore when they're feeling blue, I totally get it! We all have our thing.

Most of the time, feelings of loneliness pass quickly, but

if yours become overwhelming or don't lift after a few days, or if you find yourself feeling hopeless, losing interest in things you once loved, or experiencing suicidal thoughts, please seek help from a therapist or doctor.

Having a game plan can help you get through these times without mindlessly falling back on unhelpful or self-destructive behaviors. Try these:

- **Know your triggers**. Get real with yourself about situations when you tend to feel lonely and about how you cope. Some of your coping mechanisms might be healthy (hitting the gym, texting a supportive friend), others aren't. Resist the urge to judge or criticize yourself. Just take note.

- **Make a list of things to do when you feel lonely.** Once you've identified your triggers, come up with some alternatives. If you've noticed, for example, that Wednesday evenings are tough for you, book a weekly workout class, manicure, or other self-care practice to do something nice for yourself. If you feel especially lonely or depressed when your partner travels for work, make a date with friends to catch up while he or she is away.

    What's key about your loneliness game plan is that it needs to include activities that you actually enjoy doing (though be mindful not to make destructive choices). Don't make a list of things you think you "should" do. If cleaning when you feel down genuinely makes you feel better, awesome! But if you put "clean/organize" on the list because you're like, "I may as well do something useful if nobody wants to hang out with me," that's just going to perpetuate a self-loathing mind-set.

- **Be kind to yourself.** Changing habits is a process. It's worth noting that emotionally challenging situations can also make it harder for us to stay motivated, so if it takes some time for you to get on track with responding to loneliness constructively, that's okay. Acknowledge where you slipped up and use that information to take a better course of action next time.

What About When You Need to Grow Your Network?

If feeling like you don't have a strong network contributes to your loneliness, the good news is that it's possible to find people you connect with—yes, even as an adult.

Business coach Emily Merrell, who is the founder and chief networking officer at Six Degrees Society, used her own childhood experience of frequently changing schools as inspiration for creating a company that, as she describes it, serves as "a place where individuals could come together from all industries, all backgrounds, and show up as who they are—unapologetically. Nothing makes me happier than connecting people who could mutually make each other's lives more enjoyable."

Talking about her childhood schools, she explains that,

"The common denominator was that there was always that girl at the lunch table. You know that girl, the girl that is nice and makes an effort and takes you under her wing. She's the girl you're looking for when entering a new cafeteria, she's the one that waves you over or asks you to come over to a sleepover. She's that person that makes each day more exciting and less nervous."

Fast forward to today, says Merrell, "I'm that girl at the lunch table. I never want someone to feel the way you do on the first day at a new school at networking events. That's why I created my networking organization, Six Degrees Society."

Loneliness, she explains, is a huge problem she's trying to help solve. We're so connected and plugged in via technology "that we forget how to be alone with ourselves." What happens then is that "we start craving this external need for attention and stimulus, but we really struggle with just being." This struggle with not knowing how to enjoy our own company contributes to feeling lonely, and it's made worse, she adds, by the fear of missing out (FOMO), the comparison game, and the craving for attention and validation that social media triggers. "We need to re-teach being present," she adds, and expressing our feelings to each other.

When you move to a new city, change jobs, or when a close friend or family member moves away, these are all times you're especially vulnerable to loneliness and may benefit from going to events to help you connect with new people and expand your personal and professional network.

"I believe that it's super important to build your network when you aren't looking and tap it when you do."

Don't overlook connections you might make in line at a coffee shop or a fitness class. I met some of my closest friends waiting for the bathroom at workshops or connecting with classmates outside the fitness studio! Networking events have also been places where I've first met people who later became true friends. You just never know whom you might meet! You can also go to a structured event. Here are some of Merrell's tips for getting the most out of your networking efforts.

Show Up with an Open Mind

"Start with being open-minded and come from a place of openness," says Merrell. It can be hard to shelve expectations, but if you show up thinking you know what's going to happen, you might miss out on a great opportunity that wasn't on your radar.

Go to Events Where You'll Meet People You'd Like to Know

"Sign up for activities where you think you'd meet individuals that might convert into friendships." If you're interested in particular topics or activities and want to meet other people who enjoy those things, sign up for events centered around those things. Merrell adds, it can also help to have future events in mind if you want to ask someone to join you, so you don't feel like you're awkwardly asking, "Do you want to be friends with me?"

Go It Alone

"Don't talk yourself out of going to an event," says Merrell, because you don't have someone to go with. In fact, if you go by yourself, "you're more likely to meet people and genuinely connect with other attendees." Even if you're an introvert and this feels absolutely impossible, it's worth giving it a try.

Make the First Move

It can feel awkward, but be the one to say hi and introduce yourself. The other person will appreciate it so much—and it's a hell of a lot less awkward than just standing there making half-assed attempts at eye contact with other people. Just talk! At first it may feel uncomfortable, but over time, it gets easier, promise.

FIND A MOMENT OF PEACE
IN THE MIDDLE OF A
HECTIC DAY

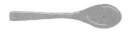

LIFE GETS BUSY and messy, and I'm always fascinated by people who say they don't have a lot of stress in their life. What is that even like? Are they just lying to themselves? Or do they know something the rest of us don't? Maybe they're kidding. Or maybe they're so used to being stressed, they don't even realize it's possible to feel better (probably the most likely).

I don't know if it's a workaholic-New-Yorker thing or a Sagittarius thing, but the second my alarm goes off in the morning, my urge is to jump up like a shot and dive head-first into my day. Some days are packed with awesome stuff, and others are packed with WTF. Usually, it's a mix. But many of us have a tendency to let the negative overpower the positive, which can color our whole week, as one day that feels like a "bad day" can trickle over into the next and so on.

While I'm all for finding ways to avoid falling into the "so-busy" trap, let's be real: no matter what your schedule or workload, finding space for peace and calm in the middle of a crazy day/week/life can be a real struggle. How do you keep it together and mellow out even when you've got a million and one things to do, or your toddler is pulling all the books off of your freshly organized shelves, or you're stuck in traffic and realize you're not going to get to that yoga class you know you really need?

While a lot depends on the situation, what I've found works for me and many of my clients is to recognize the opportunity to be mindful and find at least one positive thing to focus on in the moment. This can help us feel more peaceful and calm as we go about the rest of our day.

A lot of us feel like we get no "me" time in our day, so try reframing a challenging situation—look at a travel delay or being stuck in line at the store or on hold with customer service as the universe's way of handing you a few minutes to be with your thoughts and enjoy a little daydreaming or free-thinking.

If you're worried about running late for something like a work event (this happens to me in NYC when the subway decides to take its sweet time to arrive), contact someone at the place you need to be and let them know what's up so you're not in a panic about seeming unprofessional. Or if you're in danger of missing a connecting flight, remind yourself that staying calm will help you deal with the situation more effectively and have a better experience.

Sometimes these challenging moments can actually force us to appreciate small, good things we might normally overlook.

To share a personal example, one cold winter night (read:

huge puffy coat weather) I was stuck on a crowded, slow-dragging L-train and couldn't help getting ahead of myself worrying that it would be just as bad when I transferred to the G (another notoriously sluggish train where you get packed in like hipster sardines) to meet a guy for drinks. We'd gone out several times in the past couple months, but this time, I was sweating and freaking out ("Jess, you're really trekking way the hell from Manhattan to Brooklyn on a weeknight? You really like him. Oh no, feelings! Vulnerability!").

Then I realized that a girl I was crammed next to on the train was holding a bunch of flowers that were, in fact, right in my face. I wondered if it was her birthday or if someone had given them to her for a certain reason. Had she bought them for herself? I became invested in the story.

Because we were all pressed so close, the baby's breath in the bouquet was practically tickling my nose. I made the choice to tune way into the beautiful floral scent and the pretty pink colors. It allowed me to regroup and remind myself that staying calm would help me have a better night with the guy I was on my way to see. I also got a good laugh thinking about that literal "stop and smell the roses" parallel. Besides, when was the last time I'd been excited to the point of nervousness for a date?

He thanked me for braving the G-train.

I said, "You're on the short list of people I'll take the G for." It was the closest I'd come to showing my cards in years.

HAVE A GO-TO
CLEANSING RITUAL

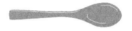

IT MAY SOUND a little woo-woo, but having a go-to cleansing ritual can help you move forward from experiences that trigger feelings of stress and anxiety. A cleansing ritual is basically something you do when you feel like you're being negatively affected by the energy around you, or when you're just feeling low or tired. Have you ever felt the need to clear lingering bad vibes in your home after a toxic roommate moved out, or to hit "reset" by getting new sheets after a breakup, or to give your ex's stuff back to them ASAP just to get it out of your space? Digital cleanses, like doing a "friend purge" on social media to cut down on political drama in your feed, count too. These are all things we might do that help us acknowledge that something happened and it affected us, but that we're choosing to move on.

I joke that bacon and nag champa (a popular type of incense with notes of sandalwood and the Champaca flower, among other resins, gums, and powders) are the scents of my childhood. Sure, we had "normal" stuff like pancakes on weekends and cold medicine in the cabinet, but we were also "the weird family" in our waspy town. For example, I didn't know anyone else whose mom was a hypnotherapist (I still don't), and while it seemed totally normal to me to talk about things like chakras and energy and to have crystals with various healing energies placed thoughtfully around the house, my friends clued me in to the fact that—nope—we were kind of . . . different.

It didn't help that we lived in what my mom's friends who worked in the paranormal and psychic healing communities described as "a very active house." I'm actually not going to write that off—growing up in a house full of weird sounds and sights instilled in me a healthy respect for the unexplainable.

My mom used to see clients in the house, and she would burn incense and sage to clear the energy. Nag champa is a scent that I'll always connect with her, as it was very warm and pleasant and it meant that she was home.

White sage, another one that was familiar to me growing up, smells a bit like marijuana, and is used for clearing negative energy or to provide protection. I have memories of my mother answering the door, saying, "I just want to let you know that even though it smells like pot, it's just sage. I was trying to clear the spirits." As a teen, I felt both mortified and proud. Another true story: The night before I left for college, my mother had me twirl around on the back porch while she waved a lit stick of white sage around me. I laughed, but it was also a very "us" moment I still keep tucked in the back of my mind. It was her way of showing me she understood and supported my wanting to shake off high school and just get on with my life.

That memory came flooding back many years later, when I was working in corporate wellness in New York. I saw patients each week in the offices of a company that was undergoing a lot of transitions, and you could practically feel the stress rippling through the organization. I got in a little early one morning, and the medical assistant was walking around with a lit stick of something that smelled familiar but slightly different.

Once she realized I was a safe person, she explained to me all about palo santo (also called "holy stick") and its energy-cleansing properties. Palo santo has been used for centuries by the Incas and indigenous peoples of the Andes for spiritual cleansing and purifying—a lovely-smelling way to chase off evil spirits.

Regardless of whether these cleansing rituals actually "work," it's been well established that scent is a powerful trigger for emotions and memories. Also, the action of taking a step to clear the energy may, in and of itself, be enough for you because, mentally, you've drawn a line in the sand and said, "I'm moving on from this uncomfortable feeling or situation and I'm burning this stick of whatever to signify that to myself."

I keep a steady supply of incense in my own home to clear anxious energy, relax, or even just mask unpleasant smells from cooking fails. I also like to use it when the seasons change or I want to mark a before/after kind of experience.

Long ago, when I lived with a roommate who disapproved of my interest in anything even slightly on the "woo" end of the spectrum, I kept a secret stash of nag champa in my desk drawer. Whenever they went out of town I'd burn it— and make sure to air out the place before they came home.

Today, it's a regular part of my self-care routine. I keep my go-to's in easy reach so it's super easy to take a few minutes out of my day to cleanse the energy.

If you decide to try this one at home, safety first! Clear away any flammable stuff like papers, and keep the lit stick of incense (or whatever you're burning) away from things like carpet and curtains. Most varieties, you use by lighting the stick or cone of incense or bundle of sage and then blowing out the flame so you get a nice little smolder. You can either walk around the space you're trying to clear, paying close attention to each corner (you might want to carry a little dish or even something like a big seashell to catch ashes in), or you can place the stick in a holder. What you choose is up to you—just be sure it's something that won't have you worrying about a lit stick falling down or blowing over.

If this sounds like way too much work, an essential oil diffuser or a candle can be an easier way to fill your space with a scent you find cleansing and comforting. Whatever approach you take, focus on what feels good to you and helps you feel centered and calm.

REWRITE THE SCRIPT

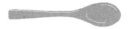

THE STORIES WE tell ourselves about who we are and what we deserve have a huge impact on our mind-set and therefore on the decisions we make.

To illustrate: Sure, I give my clients everything I've got on healthy eating strategies and self-care tips, but if they're not in a place where they truly believe that they can do it and that they deserve to feel great and meet their goals, that journey is going to be much more difficult for them.

I use that example because that's the area I work with most, but this pattern can show up in many other ways, including career, money, friendships, romantic relationships…We all have those areas where we feel confident and never worry because things just seem to flow naturally in that area. And then we have those areas where we struggle so much it hurts. Those feelings of despair, hopelessness, being overwhelmed, and being unsure of what direction to take? I've been there too.

Oftentimes, where we struggle to make progress has a

lot to do with what we tell ourselves we're capable of or even allowed to achieve. I often hear comments like, "I've tried so many diets and failed" or "I always say I'm going to get better about working out, but then I just can't stick with it." Some other common things that come up are, as we talked about previously, making negative comments about your body or about bad habits you have—like harping on your hips, thighs, or some other body part you deem imperfect, or referencing your chocolate habit. Or maybe you make excuses for yourself or try to explain away things you're not happy about. Or maybe you just tell yourself that you just have to accept the way it is.

We've talked a lot in other chapters about little hacks that can help you address the everyday issues that get in the way, but sometimes we need to go in and see where we've gotten locked into a storyline that doesn't serve us. It's a lot harder to stick to a new lifestyle change, for example, if you've been programmed to believe you're just going to fall back into old habits.

The stories we tell ourselves about how busy or stressed out we are is another loop we can get stuck on. So acknowledging which script you need to rewrite is one gigantic step. Sometimes that might take some soul-searching and maybe even some journaling. But then what?

Parijat Deshpande, MS, is a high-risk pregnancy expert and the author of *Pregnancy Brain: A Mind-Body Approach to Stress Management During a High-Risk Pregnancy*. She helps her clients identify the root causes of the stress and anxiety that trigger mental, physical, and emotional symptoms, including negative self-talk.

"Negative self-talk is a symptom of stress and anxiety and often accompanies low self-esteem," she explains. "It creates this negative feedback loop where you talk negatively to yourself and then you start to believe it and start to search for evidence that proves all the negative things you're saying about yourself."

Whether we realize it or not, we're in charge of changing that programming. Even if you can trace a problematic pattern back to someone else or to something that happened to you that was beyond your control, you have the power to rewrite your own script, and that's pretty cool.

However, rewriting your stories isn't just about doing yoga or telling yourself things you don't believe at your core.

"[Negative] self-talk is a symptom and not the root cause, so changing it doesn't make as much of a difference on stress and anxiety as we'd like to believe," Deshpande explains. Affirmations and positive self-talk alone will likely not lower heavy-duty stress and anxiety, though they can be helpful for low-grade acute stress by allowing you to take a step back and evaluate so you can approach the situation more calmly.

It's important to recognize that stress can manifest in the way our brain and body function. For example, have you ever dragged your ass to the gym after a stressful day and felt like you just didn't have the stamina you expected or wanted to have? While some people will find that the endorphins kick in and they start to feel more like themselves, some people get down on themselves about how they're never going to make progress, so why try?

Deshpande explains that cognitive issues like impaired memory and difficulty thinking clearly are very common manifestations of stress. Many people may also suffer from sleep disturbances and mental and physical fatigue. A few other big ones, as discussed in other chapters, are digestive disturbances, weight changes, and even chronic health issues like heart problems. Intense stress can also exacerbate underlying or preexisting physical and mental health issues. Because her clients are navigating fertility and pregnancy concerns, Deshpande points out that stress can also be a factor in fertility issues and pregnancy complications.

Deshpande says, a lot of times, we're conditioned to think, "'If I can think positively enough, I'll be fine, but I'm not fine, so I must not be thinking positively enough.' There's this responsibility that's placed on the self," and that self-blame can make the situation worse.

"What actually helps more," she explains, "is to identify the sources of stress and anxiety. There are often multiple factors: financial, relational, nutritional, physical pain, chronic health problems. By identifying what it is that's putting stress on your body," she explains, "it helps you see that stress is actually a physiological reaction and not just in your head, and when you can think of it that way, then you can start to see concrete steps on what to change to improve your situation.

"This gives you a sense of purpose and a clear direction of what to work on. That checklist really makes this approach very concrete and creates a sense of realistic control—not a sense of control over your entire situation. It's more, 'I have control over this piece of the situation.' You can see what those places of control are, and when you identify what you can control, that is actually the best antidote to anxiety—you can clearly see what you need to do."

While this may take some practice, she says, "you start to notice a much deeper and long-lasting shift mentally, and that shows up as the way you talk to yourself and think about your situation. The hope returns."

To share an example, I had a client who kept telling herself that she was a bad mom for not spending as much time with her son as she wanted to. She had tried writing down affirmations in her journal like, "You are a good mom," but they made her feel worse. What finally worked for her was writing down all of the things she felt were leeching her time away. Getting more clear on what she could say "no" to helped her feel more in control of her time and the stressors eating away at her. She was finally able to start spending more time with her son while still getting her work done, strengthening her belief in her parenting skills.

When to Seek Help

All of this said, if you're seriously struggling with stress and anxiety to the point where it severely disrupts your daily functioning or you're experiencing major depression or a resurfacing of health issues that require medical treatment, please seek appropriate care.

ORACLE CARDS
FOR SKEPTICS

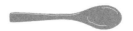

MY MOTHER GAVE me my first deck of tarot cards as a confirmation gift when I was fourteen. While my sister and I were raised Catholic, my mother encouraged us to keep the door open for spirituality in other forms. I'd shown an interest in tarot as well as in goddesses (Lilith was my favorite—it was the late 1990s and Lilith was everyone's favorite), so when she found a goddess-themed tarot deck, it couldn't have been more perfect.

A few years later, when I turned seventeen, I received a Sacred Circle deck, which is based on Celtic Paganism and features the elements and the turning of the seasons. That was my go-to deck for the next fifteen years, until a reading a friend did for me with the Wild Unknown tarot deck introduced me to a new favorite. I also have a deck of angel-themed oracle cards my mother gave me at some point when I was in college.

I'm not a tarot master—it's just an interest. Sure, I've spent way more time than I should admit nerding out on the various spreads and the suits and the minor and major arcana and definitely have certain cards I feel especially connected to, but I've never looked at tarot or oracle cards as straight-up future-telling.

What I find the cards useful for is looking at something in a way you might not have otherwise considered. In my opinion, rather than the seemingly arbitrary meaning of the card itself, the thing that tells you what you need to know is your reaction to it. This can be so helpful for digging out of an overthink-hole by getting clarity on what your gut is telling you to do, so you can move forward with a plan to help you deal with what's been wigging you out. For example, if you've been wondering about whether to look for a new job and you pull the Death card, which signifies endings and change, pay attention to the emotional response the card elicits. If your reaction is, "Phew—I feel like I have permission to walk away and look for a new job," or "Oh no—I'm not ready for this to end," that tells you a lot.

Sometimes I notice patterns where I'll draw a certain card over and over no matter how many times I shuffle the deck. For example, a card that I joke has followed me for years is the High Priestess, which is always a good reminder to trust my intuition and to set aside time to tune into it. The Nine and Ten of Cups have helped me through many an impostor syndrome slump or new relationship insecurity spiral, as they symbolize feelings of happiness and love and a sense that everything is falling into place and that it's okay to enjoy the moment. And while no one ever wants to see the Death card in their hand, it's a good reality check that endings are a natural part of life and to make room for new things, so even when it's challenging, it's still a necessary part of the big picture.

If you've never used tarot or oracle cards before, there really aren't any rules as to what the "best" option is. In general, I would just encourage choosing something that speaks to you. If this were 2003, I'd tell you to go to the New Age section of your local bookstore, but since you may not have a local bookstore anymore, check out what's popular on your favorite online retailer and see what resonates with you. Asking a friend or asking for recs "for a friend" on social media are other great ways to get suggestions.

My favorite way to use oracle cards is to take out my deck as I'm doing my morning journaling. It takes only about five minutes, but it's a ritual that helps me get into the groove of the day ahead. As I start to shuffle the cards, I ask, "What should I keep in mind today?" First, I see whether a certain card jumps or falls out at me. I also like to draw a card from the deck—no art to this, just shuffle and feel for the right card—asking, "What do I need to know?" Sometimes, I'll look at what I draw and laugh in the spirit of "tell me something I don't know," and sometimes, it won't make sense until much later in the day. If you prefer, you might draw a card in the evening and take a few minutes to reflect on the day with that message in mind.

Of course, you also have the option of being like, "Yeah, this is bullshit."

DECODE YOUR DREAMS

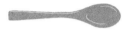

EARLIER IN THIS book we talked about hacks to help you sleep better, but what's your dream life like? Tuning into what you dream about may unlock some useful information.

Dream analysis is a therapeutic technique that's been around for thousands of years. The ancient Egyptians, for example, believed that dreams contained important messages and prophecies.

Dream analysis gained more recognition during the nineteenth century when psychotherapists began to integrate it into their work and research. It became even more widely acknowledged with the publication of Dr. Sigmund Freud's *The Interpretation of Dreams* in 1900. It was believed that dreams provided clues about our subconscious thoughts.

Regardless of whether you believe in dream analysis or not, noticing patterns in what you dream about or how your dreams make you feel can provide helpful insight into what's going on in your life.

Given that I've already blabbed about gratitude journaling, food-mood journaling, and writing down affirmations, it'll probably come as no surprise that I'm a fan of journaling about your dreams.

How to Start a Dream Journal

A dream journal practice can be as simple or as elaborate as you like. For example, when I was a teenager and had lots of free time and was bored in class, writing down my dreams in a separate notebook and spending time looking up the different symbols and their meanings in a dream dictionary was totally doable. As an adult juggling many responsibilities, writing down my dreams has become part of my morning journaling ritual. As with many practices, consistency and convenience are key.

Read Up on Symbols

Especially when it's a new practice, familiarizing yourself with common dream symbols can help you develop a basic understanding that can serve as a foundation. While it's easy to go down the rabbit hole questioning the validity and science behind it, what's really important is what certain symbols mean to *you*. As you get more comfortable with the different signs and symbols, you may find that you're able to start forming your own meaningful associations. A good starting place is an online dream dictionary. I have always been partial to Dreammoods.com, but there are so many out there, it's worth checking out a few and seeing what resonates with you.

Notice Patterns

You might think of dreaming as our mind's way of processing stuff we maybe can't or don't want to focus on in our waking life. Sometimes it can be stuff we don't even realize is taking up real estate in our brain.

Do you have the same anxiety dream all the time or notice similar themes cropping up? Do you dream about the same people or the same situations? Are your dreams stressful or do they give you valuable insight you can use? Have you noticed that you feel a certain emotion or see certain colors when you dream about a particular person? If the answer is "yes," devoting some waking time to thinking about that pattern could be valuable, as this pattern could be your brain's way of trying to focus your attention on something important to you.

Unpleasant dreams like anxiety dreams and nightmares can be especially telling. If you notice you tend to have a similar anxiety dream, that could be a sign to ask yourself what you're feeling anxious or stressed about and whether there are steps you can take to do something about it.

It's not uncommon to replay events—or variations on them—in our dreams. If those reruns are pleasant, you might tune into that happy feeling and try to come up with ways to manifest more of that in your life. However, if you're having dreams that are distressing, maybe that's pointing toward something you need to work on healing in your waking life.

WORK MEDITATION
INTO YOUR DAY

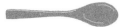

WHEN I WAS in the fifth grade, my mom decided to become a hypnotherapist. I thought it sounded interesting, but I was also afraid that someone at school would find out. After my classmates had thrown pebbles at me the year before when I'd made the mistake of talking about the ghosts in our house like it was the most normal thing (Wait, not everyone had ghosts in their house? Whoops.), I was hesitant to share anything even remotely "out there."

To make it worse, word on the playground was that our friend Brandon's dad had divorced his mom because "he found her meditating." That must have been something that the classmate who told me had overheard, because this was the '90s, and "meditation" wasn't part of our tween vocabulary. I didn't really know what meditating was, but it sure sounded scandalous.

Thankfully, my mother explained that actually, meditation wasn't a bad thing. It was basically just a way of quieting the mind through deep thinking or focusing, sometimes with chanting or someone guiding you through, sometimes in total silence. It was to help you relax or to get more in touch with your inner self—great for relieving stress and anxiety.

To call her a "hippie mama" wouldn't be quite accurate. I mean, gosh—I think she legitimately lost sleep worrying that my sister and I would try marijuana and that it would lead us down some dark path. That said, my mom practiced on us a lot of what she learned, including guided meditations and breathing techniques. There were Abraham Hicks CDs about the Law of Attraction in the car and tons of crystals scattered around the house.

When my parents had trouble selling the aforementioned haunted house, she brought in a team of "specialists" to measure the, um, activity and attempt to clear it. "You have the most *active* kitchen we've ever seen," was their assessment. It was finally a consultation with a feng shui practitioner that did the trick. You already read about how I used aromatherapy as a tool to help me on my SATs. Other people's moms hosted Tupperware parties—mine hosted meditation workshops.

Especially at that time in the 90s and early 2000s, a lot of the things that were part of my experience were considered way out there, but my mom was always very grounded in reality and tuned in to my sister and I. She also eventually became a psychotherapist so she could better support her clients.

During my teenage years, I went to a lot of wellness fairs, where I chatted up naturopaths, massage therapists, and energy healers. Some of it seemed totally legit to me, whereas some of it set off my "oh, hell no" radar. To my mother's credit, she never shoved anything down our throats, but I wanted to support her and didn't want to let anyone down.

I always tried to be respectful, even if I thought something was totally bogus, but there was this one time when I was seventeen, and I found myself sitting on the floor in a drum circle. I hadn't wanted to be there—I was at a place in my life where I really craved alone time and found other people's energy super draining, but I hadn't yet learned how to articulate my needs or protect myself from that. This circle of strangers crammed into a crowded office made me want to run and hide. I was pissed at my mom for pushing my boundaries—or maybe mad at myself for not pushing back.

Anyway, the leader of the circle beat on her drum and started shaking out her long mane of hair, asking us to channel the buffalo. *"Can you feel the buffalo?"*

I got up and walked out.

My own relationship to meditation was a bit rocky for a long time after that. I went through a (thankfully short-lived) rebellious phase in college when I turned my back on some of those wonderful things I'd been raised on: yoga, positive thinking, The Beatles . . .

I resisted meditation or anything that involved sitting still for more than a few minutes. Even when I found my way back to yoga when I moved to New York after college, I always tuned out during any chanting or meditation. I would be that person rolling up their mat and sneaking out during

Savasana. It felt too much like being a teenager forced to do something I hadn't chosen for myself.

It wasn't until I was thirty and questioning everything that I finally felt ready to establish a new relationship with meditation. Meditation apps were the thing that made it accessible enough to me to actually do it as a regular practice. I was so excited to talk to Megan Jones Bell, the Chief Science Officer at Headspace, the popular meditation app, about how to make this ancient practice approachable.

She explains that even a little can go a long way toward improving our mental state. "A lot of the research on meditation has consistently shown an impact on reducing stress and reducing anxiety, and that's also what we found in our research on Headspace," she explains. "Study after study shows a consistent effect, and I think often when you hear that, you may think it means a ton of practice, and that's actually not what we found at Headspace. A lot of the studies that we've done that have shown stress reduction or reduction in anxiety say that using our app for just ten minutes a day, about four times a week (we recommend using it daily, but we found that four times per week is about average), for anywhere from over a month to two months is where we start to see good effects for stress and anxiety reduction. We know that even after ten days, it does result in about a fourteen percent reduction of stress." She adds, "We also know that meditation changes our stress resilience pathways in the brain, changing it in a way that makes you more resilient to stress."

Meditation can also help you reframe unhelpful thoughts

or avoid going down an anxiety rabbit hole. "With stress and anxiety," she says, "our thoughts become truth without us even realizing it. They impact our emotions without us even being aware that that's what's happening. With an awareness-based practice, you're slowing that process down. You're able to see that thought arrive—whatever that anxiety or stress-provoking thought is—and with a mindful approach, you're able to recognize that it's just a thought and you're able to let it go. Essentially, it's disrupting the cycle of thoughts leading to stress and anxiety."

Want to make meditation a regular part of your life but aren't sure how to get started? Here's how.

Start Small

Jones Bell recommends, "Start by anchoring your meditation to a routine that's already well established. The example I often give is that we never think about brushing our teeth—it's just an automatic part of our morning and evening routine. How can you link a new meditation practice to something that's already on autopilot for you? Maybe after you brush your teeth, you start a three- to five-minute meditation session." Starting small like that gives you the flavor of it without the pressure of committing a huge block of time. It's also pretty hard to say you don't have three minutes for something.

Something else to try: "Maybe in those moments where you're waiting in a restaurant or you're on a bus or in a taxi you have that moment of pause." Rather than immediately whipping out your phone, says Jones Bell, "you could take a moment to focus on your breath and have that be just the very beginning of getting in your body and being aware of how your breath feels in your body."

You can gradually build up to longer meditation sessions as you feel ready and able.

Focus on Your Breath and Body

If you're having a stressful day at work, here's a tactic you can use from Jones Bell: "Concretely notice, you're sitting at your desk, having stressful thoughts. Close your eyes and focus on the breath and how it feels in your body."

You can also try a moving meditation like a walk and just focus on how your feet feel as they touch the ground. "Really simple things like that can bring you back into your body and out of your mind."

Build It into Your Schedule

If structure is helpful for you, block out the amount of time you want to meditate for. There are a ton of different answers to the question of "what's the best time of day," but especially as you're starting out, the best time is whatever time feels like the right time for you. I know tons of people who swear by a morning meditation, but after lunch can be a great time too. Or maybe for you, evening might make sense. Try out a few different times and see what feels good. Making meditation a regular part of your schedule, though, will make it a lot easier to actually do it, so you don't feel like you're trying to squeeze it in somewhere.

Meditate with Someone Else

Sometimes having someone meditate with you can help it feel more normal. "I've seen people say they wanted to try it," says Jones Bell, "and then actually do it by making it a shared practice. That can be done with friends, family, your partner, or even at work."

At the Headspace office, they have group meditation sessions twice a day, at 10 a.m. and 3 p.m. "All you have to do is walk into the room and sit down, and it eliminates that negotiation we have with ourselves because we see other people doing it, and it makes it accessible."

Jones Bell is a big believer in the power of creating a shared experience. "Meditation was something that previously I had done solo, and it was through experiencing our work environment, where we have these well-attended group meditation experiences, [that it felt like I was] part of something." There's also the benefit of increased focus afterward. "It feels like when I go back into my back-to-back meetings, I'm much more deliberate, I'm much more present, and I'm still energized, but I'm more clear and focused, and I'm very intentional, and it's a lot easier to be present."

Let Go of the "Empty Mind" Ideal

Yes, meditation can be powerful tool to declutter gunk that's in your brain, but it's completely normal to become aware of thoughts that flutter to the front of your mind when you're meditating.

And if you feel yourself starting to get stressed out by those thoughts, says Jones Bell, "There's not something wrong with you! Accept that our mind takes us places that sometimes aren't very helpful for us to go."

However, she adds, cultivating an enhanced awareness of your thoughts through a meditation practice can actually help you spot those thoughts that could send you on a stress spiral and empower you to "step alongside them. You may not be able to reverse them, but you can step alongside them and say, 'I'm going down that rabbit hole.' Bringing awareness to your body is a great way of disrupting your stress response. Focusing on your breath and activating your relaxation response can help unglue those thoughts in your mind."

Meditation, she explains, is "not about distracting. It's about redirecting our attention to our body as opposed to those stressful thoughts. It's a helpful way of releasing those thoughts instead of getting attached to them."

LET GO OF FOOD GUILT

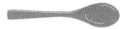

I'M FORTUNATE ENOUGH to work with wonderful, amazing clients and to interview successful, brilliant people who are at the top of their field, and I'm struck by how many of them experience or have struggled with feeling guilty about what they eat.

While it's totally human and normal to be, like, "Okay, I don't feel so great after eating that," heavy-duty food guilt, especially when it gets tied in to feelings of self-worth, can drag us down in many areas of our life.

Negative self-talk, which we've discussed previously, can distract us from other things that need our energy and attention. If you've ever tried to focus on work when the voice in your head was sneering at you (*Why did you eat that? You're disgusting.*) then you know what I'm talking about. When we feel guilty, it also can cause us to criticize or punish ourselves by making choices that don't support our goals. Guilt is an energy-sucking emotion that negatively influences how we feel about ourselves and how we interact with others around us. It also chips away at our self-esteem, which can make it hard to feel motivated to invest in ourselves and make choices that support our overall wellness. For example, if you feel guilty about something you ate earlier in the day, you might have a harder time feeling confident about your ability to make a positive choice at your next eating occasion.

Here are some of the approaches I take with my clients to help them let go of food guilt.

Know What Triggers You

We're all different, and that's okay. The foods and situations that cause one person to spiral down into food guilt may be no big deal to someone else. And these triggers can be specific—maybe you feel like you can't be around pizza without overindulging in it, but feel no guilt around the regular Sunday pancakes you enjoy with your family.

Oftentimes these are learned behaviors. For example, if you were brought up in a home where everyone was always on a diet or there was a lot of talk about how unhealthy certain foods were, you may struggle as an adult with guilt around eating those things. It's not uncommon to have a hard time being moderate with "forbidden fruit" items, or to feel like you have to bash yourself for enjoying a treat.

Of course, we can also pick up messages from our friends and colleagues. When the people around us are following a certain regimen or swearing off a particular food (or food category, like sugar), it's easy to feel pressured to follow suit, even if no one directly says anything to you. That pressure often stems from wanting to feel like part of a group or from self-doubt that manifests in a lack of confidence in our food choices.

When my clients ask me if they should be drinking apple cider vinegar or whether carbs are going to make them fat or if they should do a juice cleanse, my first question is usually, "What made you interested in that?" Similarly, if someone expresses feeling guilt for eating a particular food, we talk about where they think that might be coming from.

While we may not be able to control all of the triggers we encounter, we do hold sway over how we respond to them. Cultivating awareness of the situations in which we're most prone to feeling guilty empowers us to recognize when we're about to go down that path and redirect our thoughts to something more constructive.

Be Careful with Social Media

What we see in our social media feeds can have a huge impact on how we feel about ourselves, and that, in turn, may influence the choices we make about our health, food, and fitness. Surround yourself with images and messages that make you feel good, and avoid the ones that make you feel pressured to adhere to an impossible standard or that make you feel less-than.

One of my favorite expressions is "compare and despair" because it's just so true. When we compare our internal blooper reel to the highlight reels we see all around us, it's a losing game. Even though we know, logically, that people curate, it's hard to keep that at the top of our mind when we're in the middle of scrolling.

For example, if you feel guilty for eating a donut for breakfast after you see a post of a vegan smoothie bowl on Instagram, and will punish yourself with an extra-long run or by skipping lunch, you just got a very clear sign to unfollow that account.

The chapter on the power of intention with Lisa Skye Hain delves more into how following social media accounts that make us feel uplifted and inspired can foster a more positive, can-do mind-set. You want that time you spend scrolling to help you feel inspired, not inferior.

Focus on What Makes You Feel Good

It's so easy to fixate on what you did "wrong," but I encourage my clients to instead focus on what makes them feel good. Rather than thinking you have to make up for "bad" behavior or punish yourself, set an intention to move forward by enjoying foods and activities that help you feel well.

To go back to the donut example, if you ate a donut for breakfast, take a moment to note what you enjoyed about it. It's normal to have some negative thoughts about it, so if those float to the surface, acknowledge them and then let them go. Sure, it might not be the most nutritious way to start your day, but what enjoyment or positivity did it offer you, and why was that important? Then, rather than chastising yourself, simply plan to have a protein-rich lunch with lots of vegetables to help you get your blood sugar and energy on track and to get some important nutrients into your day.

If you wake up feeling like crap after an indulgent night out, you can file away that feeling as motivation not to have that third drink next time, but then don't starve yourself and try to sweat away your sins at a balls-to-the-wall bootcamp class or whatever you think you're supposed to do to atone. Drink a tall glass of water, enjoy a balanced breakfast, and set an intention to enjoy whatever type of movement your body is asking for that day—or to rest, if that's what you need.

Be Patient with Yourself

Unlearning food guilt is a process that takes time. Be patient with yourself. It gets easier with practice to spot when you need to let go of guilt, but if you do find yourself caught in the current of food guilt, you haven't failed. You're working on building a new pattern, and even the times you struggle can teach you something.

Take a deep breath and give yourself permission to move on mindfully. A mantra I often have my clients repeat to themselves is, "You are making steady progress." Because this is often such a private struggle, you may not feel like you have a lot of positive reinforcement when you need it. Reminding yourself of how well you're doing can help you keep at it.

Just a side note: If you feel that your food guilt is having a severe impact on your quality of life, seek help from a therapist or dietitian. While the techniques discussed above can help, working one-on-one with an appropriate professional may be necessary when you're really struggling.

LOSE THE LABELS

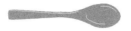

SOMETHING THAT SOMETIMES freaks out my new clients is when I encourage them to ditch the labels they assign to their diet.

So many people are so used to having a name for the diet they follow, the idea of not having that as a framework can be scary. Rather than seeing the freedom in eating what feels right for them and their body without a Vegan/Vegetarian/Keto/Paleo/[whatever the hell is trending this week] categorization, they panic. What if not having any limits becomes a free-for-all?

The good news is that almost everyone comes to love having the flexibility to choose based on their unique needs. Here are some basic tips to help you get started with becoming a flexible eater.

Journal It Out
If you're new to the concept of eating whatever you want without that being a "bad" thing, journaling can be incredibly valuable in helping you tune into which foods help you

feel great and which foods and combinations just don't do it for you. Remember, this should be about you and you alone—not how you think you should be eating or how someone else wants you to eat.

As patterns start to emerge or you notice changes or shifts you need to make, go with it. The body is really smart and will tell us what it needs—we just have to listen. As I talked about in earlier chapters, my cravings for high-fat foods like sardines packed in olive oil were a clue to me that my stress levels were insanely high and that I needed to take a holistic approach to get a handle on that. Or say you eat mainly plant protein but get an intense craving for steak out of seemingly nowhere, it could be a sign that your iron is a little low and your body is asking for help replenishing its stores.

If your cravings are freaking you out, reach out to your doctor and ask whether there are any medical tests that could rule out an underlying problem.

Make It Easy

Once you know what you need to feel great, make it convenient to make it happen. Stock up on the basics you need and plan ahead if you know you're going to be really busy. If it'll make you feel better, or if the shifts you're allowing yourself to make impact other people you're living with or share meals with regularly, you can let them know.

Give Yourself Permission to Change

What works for us at one time in our life can change. Check in with yourself along the way. To share a personal example, when I was in my twenties, I ate sweet oatmeal for breakfast pretty much every day. Then when I was twenty-seven, I suddenly got a taste for savory breakfast and savory oats became a regular thing. Then when I was thirty-one, I suddenly couldn't stand the thought of oatmeal or grains in general. I made sure to cover my nutritional bases, but because I felt really good starting my day with things like eggs, vegetables, and potatoes, I didn't bother to look back. I figure that throughout my life, I'll continue to go through changes in what feels good as my body chemistry changes, and I'm okay with that.

Bottom Line

Ditching the labels around what you eat can help you better connect with your body and what you need to thrive.

BREAK THAT PATTERN.
YOU KNOW THE ONE.

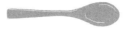

WE ALL HAVE a habit or pattern that feels impossible to break. We know it's not helping us—maybe it's even bad for us—but awareness that this is our "thing" just doesn't seem to be enough to get us to move on.

I spoke with Karen Noé, a New Jersey-based psychic medium, spiritual counselor, and healer with a two-year waiting list. She is also the author of books such as *We Consciousness*, *Your Life After Their Death*, and *Through the Eyes of Another*. She helps her clients find healing through her readings and classes as well as her radio show and writing.

Much of her work centers on the Law of Attraction and on cultivating a positive outlook and loving energy. Changing a behavior, breaking a habit, and establishing a new pattern all take some inner work so you can move forward in a positive direction. Here's how.

Look Inside
Being aware of the issue you want to work on is a good starting place, but it helps to understand where it comes

from if you're having trouble breaking an old pattern or you want to gain clarity on your problematic relationship with a particular person or thing.

There are many ways of tuning in. Journaling or meditation are a few things you can try solo. Talking with a therapist can also be incredibly helpful. Noticing patterns or trends that stick out and putting together an origin story of sorts can help you catch yourself when you're starting to act or respond in that unhelpful way.

You could also try a past life regression, a form of hypnosis used to tap into memories from a past incarnation, to see how old patterns and relationships might be playing out in this current life. Whether you actually believe in past lives or not doesn't really matter, but you're getting insight into your emotional truth so you can use that information to make changes or approach a situation differently. Even if you don't believe in past life regression, you could look at it as insight into your emotional history with a particular person or situation, or as a way to highlight an emotion you may not have been clued into before. For example, if you "starved to death in a past life," it could shed some light on issues with compulsive eating or your fear of food scarcity.

Cleanse and Protect

Noé uses cleansing rituals as a daily essential. One of her favorites is the "Celtic weave," a technique popularized by *Energy Medicine* author Donna Eden, she explains, in which you move your arms in formations meant to help weave the energy around you so you're protected from negative energy you might encounter. She also regularly burns sage and incense and diffuses essential oils to cleanse and protect her workspace and living space. If she's burning sage, she'll also use sweetgrass. "The sage takes away the negative energy and the sweetgrass puts in positive energy. It's not just about removing the negative—it's also about making the room feel good."

If your loved ones aren't open to the idea of cleansing rituals, she says, "you don't even have to tell them what you're doing." If you're doing something like the weave, you can do it before you go out for the day, or in the bathroom if you're with others.

Another great way to cleanse, Noé shares, is to clean out your physical space. That can be giving away things you don't need, rearranging furniture to feel more harmonious, and opening the windows to let some fresh air into the room—and your life. That fresh air and extra room can help you feel like you can breathe more easily and think more clearly, which can be helpful when trying to make a change in your habits.

Set an Intention

"It's all about energy," explains Noé. "We're vibrational beings. Whatever we're thinking and feeling, we're creating more of that in our lives. Whatever that dominant feeling is—if it's a feeling of positivity, we're creating more positive energy. If it's negativity, we're creating more negative energy." Even if you're saying, "I don't want this," she explains, by focusing on that thing you don't want, you're still drawing it to you.

She says, "The bottom line is: Focus on what you do want instead of what you don't want. Focus on the solutions instead of the problems. Focus on the blessings instead of on what's wrong. It's not always easy, you have to learn how to do that."

One powerful exercise Noé does with her clients is to have them state a goal or intention. For example, "By this time next year, I will have_____ in my life." She has them name the things that they want to manifest in their life. You can write out your intentions or declare them out loud—the power comes from repetition. Try it in the morning and evening daily and prepare to be amazed at what transpires. "Even if you don't have the faith in that happening, fake it until you make it and keep saying it. In thirty days, you will feel different and you will be amazed at the opportunities and people who come into your life, and you will know you actually made it happen."

Worried that you won't be able to break a bad habit? "I would also say fake it until you make it," says Noé. She's a big believer in positive affirmations. "Say it until you believe it." One she uses with a lot of her clients is, "I am open and receptive to everything around me. I am open and receptive to the many blessings in the world." When you do that, she explains, "you're shifting your vibration, you're shifting your negative thoughts," which can help you turn challenges you're going through into something positive. This can help you feel more confident in your ability to change and may make it easier for you to adopt new, positive habits.

Monitor Your Feelings

We often hear about monitoring our thoughts, but that can be overwhelming for people who feel like their thoughts move way too fast for them to keep track of.

Noé encourages her clients to focus on their feelings instead. "You can't monitor every single one of your thoughts because they go a mile a minute, but what you can monitor is your feelings within you. If you're feeling positive, you're thinking positive thoughts, and if you're feeling down in the dumps, chances are you're thinking more negative thoughts."

There are lots of ways to shift your energy from negative to positive. "You can look up videos of things that make you laugh," says Noé, who says that YouTube clips of cute animals and of babies laughing helped her get through a divorce. "You can also put on music, go for a walk—whatever works for you."

She also has clients play what she calls the "Yes, But" game, in which you note that something negative happened but add one positive thing. For example, maybe you're devastated over losing your job, but now you have time to see friends and family you may have felt disconnected from when you were busting your ass nonstop. That sets the stage to explore other positive outcomes stemming from what you're going through.

Tune into Gratitude

There are going to be times when we might not feel like we have anything to be grateful for. This is where making gratitude a regular part of your routine can be a game changer. You can start with the basics, says Noé. "First thing in the morning when you open your eyes, before you even get out of bed, say something you're grateful for." It could be something as simple as "the bed I'm sleeping in," or "having heat and hot water."

You can also practice saying "thank you" for small, good things throughout the day: a delicious cup of coffee, the subway train appearing right after you reach the platform, a positive interaction with a colleague—whatever you like. Noé's "Yes, But" game can also be a helpful way to put a positive spin on day-to-day challenges that come up.

Over time, this helps make a positive mind-set your resting state—or at least much easier to tap into! As you build new habits and tweak what you need to along the way, you'll gradually become more conscious of what you want to perpetuate in your daily life.

EMBRACE THE MAGIC
OF DECLUTTERING

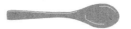

SEVERAL OF THE experts I spoke with in other chapters have already talked about the magic of cleaning out our physical space as a means of clearing the mind, but there's a reason I'm devoting an entire chapter to this topic: it freaking works.

If you've never tried this one, put it on your *must*-do list. By cleaning up and organizing our physical surroundings, it makes space for things we want to welcome into our life and helps us be in a more clearheaded mind-set to receive them.

As Karen Noé spoke about in the chapter about cleansing rituals, getting rid of things we no longer need and want is a healthy sign that we're ready to move on to a new phase. Feeling like we have more physical space can also help us feel less stressed out if we struggle with feeling stuck or stagnant or claustrophobic in a current pattern.

Whenever my clients tell me their weekend plans include cleaning out their closet, or doing a deep clean of their apartment, I can tell they're making meaningful progress with settling into a healthier new pattern. That could be something like getting rid of clothes that don't fit or that they don't feel great in, or as one of my clients did, turning a cluttered guest room into a retreat where she could journal and meditate and stream yoga classes on her laptop!

Sometimes the act of letting go of physical stuff can ease us into important transitions. Over the years, I've noticed in my own life that big shifts happen in my love life when I empty out shelves and drawers and dust under the bed.

Years ago, for example, I was living with a boyfriend in midtown Manhattan. Our lease was going to be up in July, and we lived in a part of town that had started to feel chaotic and cramped, so we started exploring other parts of the city. We almost applied for a few, but then one morning he woke up and said, "I want to stay here." It was the summer we had eight (yes, eight) weddings to go to, and the argument that we'd be spending a lot of time and money traveling and purchasing gifts was compelling. So we did a "deep clean" where we literally pulled all the furniture into the middle of the room, dusted and washed every corner and crevice, and gave away a ton of things we no longer used. We rearranged the furniture.

I had hoped that the apartment would feel more welcoming afterward, but the strain only got worse. Since he usually got home later than I did, I used to listen for his key in the lock and cringe when I heard the click. On weekends we were local, I wandered the city by myself or made plans with friends while he stayed home on the computer with his headphones on.

All these years later, I honestly feel like that deep clean was part of that mental shift that helped us pull away from each other without there needing to be any big event that tore out the sutures. Of course, there's also the fact that going to eight weddings and watching friends and family declare "Until death do us part" makes you question what the hell you're doing and whether that's a choice you should make.

That's why I didn't question it when, after my father died, the only thing I wanted to do for weeks was clean. For the fifteen months that he'd been sick, I'd basically been phoning it in with my cleaning and decluttering efforts—and feeling disconnected from myself and the other people in my life. I was in a rut. A thin film of dust covered nearly every surface of my apartment, and suddenly I could see how my closet was packed with clothes I hadn't touched in years, making it hard to find what I actually wanted to wear. I felt like I couldn't breathe. I felt like I had nothing to wear and had no idea how to get into a new pattern.

I started with my shoes. Then I moved onto the coats. How can one person have so many? I donated books and household goods and shredded so. much. paper. I also burned a ton of palo santo. Within a week of my cleansing adventure, I felt like a new person. For the first time in over a year, I could name what I wanted and how I planned to make it a reality. Interestingly, those things began to show up, as if by magic. The path began to reveal itself, and in better, more exciting ways than I could have dreamed.

If you want to try this out for yourself, here are a few tips.

Start Small

If your big goal is to clean and declutter your whole home or even a whole room, don't put the pressure on yourself to climb that mountain all in one go. Start super small. As Leanne Jacobs said in the chapter about manifestation, even just sorting through the drawer where you keep bills and paying a few can help you feel calmer.

Set Guidelines

If structure helps you feel calmer, set yourself a schedule of what you're going to work on and in what order or on what days. If you're undertaking a project like going through your closet, if you need to, set yourself some rules to make it easier to know what to toss. For example, if you haven't worn it in x number of months or if it makes you feel miserable or brings up bad memories, that's a clue to get rid of it. If you're like me and sometimes stumble on a box of old papers from college or grad school, ask yourself if you've ever once reached for those materials or anticipate ever needing them. Also, I know that sentimentality is strong, but never underestimate the satisfaction of shredding an old love letter from someone whose memory makes your blood boil. You'll wonder what took you so long.

Enlist Help if Needed

There's no shame in hiring a professional if you just can't face the task alone. A professional organizer or a cleaning service can work magic. Of course, you can also call in friends and family members you know will be able to give you honest, constructive input as you sort and sift.

Practice Mindful (Re)Placement

If you're doing any rearranging of furniture or purchasing new items to replace things you've let go of, be mindful and intentional about where you put your new acquisitions. Arranging furniture and items based on how you use them can add a sense of ease to your day. For example, you could place a chair near the closet where you keep your shoes so you can sit comfortably while you put them on in the morning. Or in the kitchen, set up the blender on your counter near things you use every day to make a smoothie. The goal is to streamline your day-to-day movements in a way that will bring joy to your mind, body, and spirit.

Bottom Line

Cleaning and organizing your physical space is a powerful way to shift your mind-set and make space for what you want to manifest. Try it.

SO NOW WHAT?

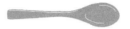

I WISH I could tell you—and myself—that now that you've finished this book, you will never experience stress again, that you will never struggle with work-life balance, that every single goal you set will be a breeze, or that you will never fall into the comparison trap when you're having a tough day. The annoying truth, of course, is that there are always going to be barriers to work through—uncomfortable situations that come up and threaten to knock us off balance. It's part of the human experience.

What I can tell you is that you have many tools and resources at your disposal, and most of them are within you. My hope is that you'll be able to take the game changers in this book and put them to work for you, so that you can more easily stay on a path that feels good and brings a sense of ease back into your life.

When you feel yourself struggling, go back to those vital signs we talked about in the first chapter. Check in with yourself about your:

Energy
Anxiety
Stress
Emotions

As you go down the list, do a little check-in. How do you feel? What's causing you to feel that way? What feels in balance? What feels out of balance? What's working? What's not? What can you control? What's out of your hands? Which game changers can help you feel like you're more able to stand your ground or move in the direction you want to? Revisit that work-life balance pie chart if you need to.

At different times in our lives, we'll find that we need to reevaluate and adjust our strategies. Some days we're going to feel more successful than others, and that's okay. When you need to get back in balance or back on track toward a goal, lean in to those tiny tweaks you *can* make. Don't be afraid to start small. Those microscopic shifts can have a big impact. Also, remember to acknowledge your progress along the way.

Fad diets and fitness trends will come and go, but at the end of the day, you're the expert on you, and your body is really smart—listen to it.

ACKNOWLEDGMENTS

THIS BOOK WOULD not be possible without the support of so many people.

I want to start by thanking my family. I'm so lucky to have been raised by two amazing parents who encouraged me to follow my heart and to not be afraid to work hard doing what I love. I'm also grateful to have a great sister on this adventure with me.

Another big thank you to Jacob Tschetter, for your loving kindness. I'm not sure how I would have gotten through this process without your pep talks, reality checks, and home-made green juice and cocktails.

Thank you to my wonderful agent, Leigh Eisenman, for your guidance and support.

I am so grateful to the wonderful team at Viva Editions, especially to my editor, Hannah Bennett, and to Allyson Fields, for believing in the book and helping me see the project through. Thank you to my publicist, Kathleen Carter for helping us take that vision further.

Thank you to the experts quoted in this book who were so generous with their time and insight: Megan Jones Bell, Dr. Taz Bhatia, Lauren Chiarello, Parijat Deshpande, Annbeth Eschbach, Ashley Feinstein Gerstley, Lisa Skye Hain, Leanne Jacobs, Dr. Sujay Kinsagra, Johari Mayfield, Emily Merrell, Mandi Nyambi, Karen Noé, and Ryan Smith. I'm so grateful to have learned from you. Additionally, I want to express my gratitude to the outlets I have written for and organizations I have worked with through which I met some many of these experts.

Special thanks to my earliest test readers, Arissa Paschalidis, Mike Smith, and Cory Bradburn. Additional thank you to Armin Brott for helping me tighten up the manuscript.

I want to acknowledge my friends for their support, encouragement, and advice. Lemor Balter, Amanda Dugan, Alex Dickinson, Jess Garofano, Elana Lyn Gross, Brian Hodges, Anders and Carrie Nelson, Jill Ozovek, Dan Schawbel, and Devany Tiedman.

I also want to give a shout out to my friends in the yoga, barre, and Pilates communities for saving my posture (and my sanity) while I worked on this book—and for brightening my days with their warmth and energy.

ENDNOTES

1   "Vital Signs (Body Temperature, Pulse Rate, Respiration Rate, Blood Pressure)," Johns Hopkins Medicine. https://www. hopkinsmedicine.org/health/conditions-and-diseases/vital-signs-body-temperature-pulse-rate-respiration-rate-blood-pressure.

2   "Stress," Anxiety and Depression Association of America, ADAA. https://adaa.org/understanding-anxiety/related-illnesses/ stress.

3   "5 Things You Should Know About Stress," National Institute of Mental Health. https://www.nimh.nih.gov/health/publications/stress/index.shtml.

4   Ashish Sharma, Vishal Madaan, and Frederick D. Petty. "Exercise for Mental Health." *The Journal of Clinical Psychiatry.* https:// www.ncbi.nlm.nih.gov/pmc/articles/PMC1470658/.

5   "Positive Emotions and Your Health: Developing a Brighter Outlook," *News in Health*, August 2015. https://newsinhealth. nih.gov/2015/08/positive-emotions-your-health.

6   Claire Eagleson, Sarra Hayes, Andrew Mathews, Gemma Perman, and Colette R. Hirsch, "The Power of Positive Thinking: Pathological Worry Is Reduced by Thought Replacement in Generalized Anxiety Disorder," *Behaviour Research and Therapy* 78 (March 2016): 13–18. doi:10.1016/j.brat.2015.12.017. https://www.ncbi.nlm.nih.gov/pmc/articles/PMC4760272/.

7   "Daily Life," The American Institute of Stress. https://www. stress.org/daily-life.

8   "Brain Reward Pathways," Icahn School of Medicine | Neuroscience Department | Nestler Lab | Brain Reward Pathways. https://

neuroscience.mssm.edu/nestler/brainRewardpathways.html.

9 "Aromatherapy with Essential Oils," National Cancer Institute. https://www.cancer.gov/about-cancer/treatment/cam/patient/aromatherapy-pdq?redirect=true.

10 Y. Soudry, C. Lemogne, D. Malinvaud, S.-M. Consoli, and P. Bonfils, "Olfactory System and Emotion: Common Substrates," *European Annals of Otorhinolaryngology, Head and Neck Diseases* 128, no. 1 (January 11, 2011): 18–23. doi:10.1016/j.anorl.2010.09.007. https://www.ncbi.nlm.nih.gov/pubmed/21227767.

11 *Lavender.* Bethesda, MD: National Center for Complementary and Integrative Health, 2008. https://nccih.nih.gov/health/lavender/ataglance.htm.

12 *Peppermint Oil.* Bethesda, MD: National Center for Complementary and Integrative Health, 2008. https://nccih.nih.gov/health/peppermintoil.

13 Mark Moss, Steven Hewitt, Lucy Moss, and Keith Wesnes, "Modulation of Cognitive Performance and Mood by Aromas of Peppermint and Ylang-Ylang," *International Journal of Neuroscience* 118, no. 1 (January 2008): 59–77. doi:10.1080/00207450601042094. https://www.ncbi.nlm.nih.gov/pubmed/18041606.

14 Dalina Isabel, Sanchez-Vidana, Shirley Pui-Ching Ngai, Wanjia He, Jason Ka-Wing Chow, Benson Wui-Man Lau, and Hector Wing-Hong Tsang, "The Effectiveness of Aromatherapy for Depressive Symptoms: A Systematic Review," *Evidence-Based Complementary and Alternative Medicine* 2017 (January 2017): 1–21. doi:10.1155/2017/5869315. https://www.ncbi.nlm.nih.gov/pmc/articles/PMC5241490/.

15 Sanchez-Vidana, et al. "The Effectiveness of Aromatherapy for Depressive Symptoms," 1-21.

16 Safieh Mohebitabar, Mahboobeh Shirazi, Sodabeh Bioos, Roja Rahimi, Farhad Malekshahi, and Fatemeh Nejatbakhsh, "Therapeutic Efficacy of Rose Oil: A Comprehensive Review of Clinical Evidence," *Avicenna Journal of Phytomedicine* (May-June 2017): 206–13. https://www.ncbi.nlm.nih.gov/pmc/articles/ PMC5511972/.

17 Winai Sayorwan, et al. "Effects of Inhaled Rosemary Oil on Subjective Feelings and Activities of the Nervous System," *Scientia Pharmaceutica*81, no. 2 (April 2013): 531–42. December 23, 2012. doi:10.3797/scipharm.1209-05. https:// www.ncbi.nlm.nih.gov/pmc/articles/PMC3700080/.

18 CDC - Frequently Asked Questions - Alcohol. Centers for Disease Control and Prevention. https://www.cdc.gov/alcohol/ faqs.htm.

19 Hong-Xing Wang, and Yu-Ping Wang, "Gut Microbiota-brain Axis," *Chinese Medical Journal* 129, no. 19 (October 5, 2016): 2373–380. doi:10.4103/0366-6999.190667. https://www.ncbi. nlm.nih.gov/pmc/articles/PMC5040025/.

20 John B Furness, Brid P. Callaghan, Leni R. Rivera, and Hyun-Jung Cho, "The Enteric Nervous System and Gastrointestinal Innervation: Integrated Local and Central Control," *Advances in Experimental Medicine and Biology Microbial Endocrinology: The Microbiota-Gut-Brain Axis in Health and Disease*, 2014, 39–71. doi:10.1007/978-1-4939-0897-4_3. https://www.ncbi.nlm. nih.gov/pubmed/24997029.

21 Helen Fields, "The Gut: Where Bacteria and Immune System Meet," Johns Hopkins Medicine, Baltimore, Maryland. November 2015. https://www.hopkinsmedicine.org/research/ advancements-in-research/fundamentals/in-depth/the-gut-where-bacteria-and-immune-system-meet.

22 "What Happens When Your Immune System Gets Stressed Out?" Health Essentials from Cleveland Clinic. March 3, 2015.

https://health.clevelandclinic.org/what-happens-when-your-immune-system-gets-stressed-out/.

23 Katherine Zeratsky, RD "What Are Probiotics and Prebiotics?" Mayo Clinic. June 28, 2018. https://www.mayoclinic.org/healthy-lifestyle/consumer-health/expert-answers/probiotics/faq-20058065.

24 Venera Cardile, et al. "Gelatin Tannate Reduces the Proinflammatory Effects of Lipopolysaccharide in Human Intestinal Epithelial Cells," *Clinical and Experimental Gastroenterology 61*, May 8, 2012, doi:10.2147/CEG.S28792. https://www.ncbi.nlm.nih.gov/pmc/articles/PMC3358810/.

25 Guoyao Wu, Fuller W. Bazer, et al. "Proline and Hydroxyproline Metabolism: Implications for Animal and Human Nutrition," *Amino Acids* 40, no. 4 (August 10, 2010): 1053–63. doi:10.1007/s00726-010-0715-z. https://www.ncbi.nlm.nih.gov/pmc/articles/PMC3773366/.

26 Xiao Xu, Xiuying Wang, et al. "Glycine Relieves Intestinal Injury by Maintaining mTOR Signaling and Suppressing AMPK, TLR4, and NOD Signaling in Weaned Piglets after Lipopolysaccharide Challenge," *International Journal of Molecular Sciences* 19, no. 7 (July 06, 2018): 1980. doi:10.3390/ijms19071980. https://www.ncbi.nlm.nih.gov/pmc/articles/PMC6073676/.

27 Radha Krishna Rao and Geetha Samak. "Role of Glutamine in Protection of Intestinal Epithelial Tight Junctions," *Journal of Epithelial Biology and Pharmacology* 5, no. 1 (August 22, 2011): 47–54. doi:10.2174/1875044301205010047. https://www.ncbi.nlm.nih.gov/pmc/articles/PMC4369670/.

28 Qianru Chen, Oliver Chen, Isabela M. Martins, Hu Hou, Xue Zhao, Jeffrey B. Blumberg, and Bafang Li. "Collagen Peptides Ameliorate Intestinal Epithelial Barrier Dysfunction in Immunostimulatory Caco-2 Cell Monolayers via Enhancing Tight Junctions," *Food & Function* 8, no. 3 (March 22, 2017):

1144–151. doi:10.1039/c6foo1347c. https://www.ncbi.nlm.nih.gov/pubmed/28174772.

29 Gunaranjan Paturi, Christine A. Butts, and Kerry L. Bentley-Hewitt, "Influence of Dietary Avocado on Gut Health in Rats," *Plant Foods for Human Nutrition* 72, no. 3 (September 2017): 321–23. doi:10.1007/s11130-017-0614-5. https://www.ncbi.nlm.nih.gov/pubmed/28550342.

30 Isabel Prieto, et al, "Influence of a diet enriched with virgin olive oil or butter on mouse gut microbiota and its correlation to physiological and biochemical parameters related to metabolic syndrome," January 2018. https://doi.org/10.1371/journal.pone.0190368.

31 "Why Stress Causes People to Overeat," *Harvard Health Publishing*, February 2012. https://www.health.harvard.edu/staying-healthy/why-stress-causes-people-to-overeat.

32 "Choline Fact Sheet for Health Professionals." NIH Strengthening Knowledge and Understanding of Dietary Supplements. https://ods.od.nih.gov/factsheets/Choline-HealthProfessional/.

33 "Folate Fact Sheet for Health Professionals," NIH Strengthening Knowledge and Understanding of Dietary Supplements. https://ods.od.nih.gov/factsheets/Folate-HealthProfessional/.

34 "Calcium Fact Sheet for Health Professionals," NIH Strengthening Knowledge and Understanding of Dietary Supplements. https://ods.od.nih.gov/factsheets/Calcium-HealthProfessional/.

35 Beata Olas, "Berry Phenolic Antioxidants–Implications for Human Health?" *Frontiers in Pharmacology* 9 (March 26, 2018). doi:10.3389/fphar.2018.00078. https://www.ncbi.nlm.nih.gov/pmc/articles/PMC5890122/.

36 Grace E. Giles, Caroline R. Mahoney, Heather L. Urry, Tad T. Brunyé, Holly A. Taylor, and Robin B. Kanarek, "Omega-3 Fatty Acids and Stress-Induced Changes to Mood and Cognition in Healthy Individuals." *Pharmacology Biochemistry and Behavior* 132 (May 2015): 10–19. doi:10.1016/j.pbb.2015.02.018. https://www.ncbi.nlm.nih.gov/pubmed/25732379.

37 Jedha Dening, "Role of Olive Oil in Reducing Oxidative Stress," *Olive Oil Times*, June 8, 2016. https://www.oliveoiltimes.com/olive-oil-basics/role-olive-oil-reducing-oxidative-stress/50816.

38 Adrian L. Lopresti, "Efficacy of Curcumin, and a Saffron/Curcumin Combination for the Treatment of Major Depression: A Randomised, Double-Blind, Placebo-Controlled Study," *Journal of Affective Disorders* 207 (January 2017): 188–96. doi:10.1016/j.jad.2016.09.047. https://www.ncbi.nlm.nih.gov/m/pubmed/27723543/.

39 Ahmed Al Sunni, and Rabia Latif, "Effects of Chocolate Intake on Perceived Stress: A Controlled Clinical Study," *International Journal of Health Sciences* 8, no. 4 (October 2014): 393–401. doi:10.12816/0023996. https://www.ncbi.nlm.nih.gov/pmc/articles/PMC4350893/.

40 Janice K. Kiecolt-Glaser. "Stress, Food, and Inflammation: Psychoneuroimmunology and Nutrition at the Cutting Edge," *Psychosomatic Medicine* 72, no. 4 (May 2010): 365–69. doi:10.1097/psy.0b013e3181dbf489. https://www.ncbi.nlm.nih.gov/pmc/articles/PMC2868080/.

41 "Dietary Fats," American Heart Association. https://www.heart.org/en/healthy-living/healthy-eating/eat-smart/fats/dietary-fats.

42 Laurence Eyres, Michael F. Eyres, Alexandra Chisholm, and Rachel C. Brown, "Coconut Oil Consumption and Cardiovascular Risk Factors in Humans," *Nutrition Reviews* 74, no. 4

(March 05, 2016): 267–80. doi:10.1093/nutrit/nuw002. https://www.ncbi.nlm.nih.gov/pmc/articles/PMC4892314/.

43   "Omega-3 Fatty Acids Fact Sheet for Health Professionals," NIH Strengthening Knowledge and Understanding of Dietary Supplements. https://ods.od.nih.gov/factsheets/Omega3Fatty-Acids-HealthProfessional/.

44 Philip C. Clader, "Omega-3 Fatty Acids and Inflammatory Processes," *Nutrients* 2, no. 3 (March 18, 2010): 355–74. doi:10.3390/nu2030355.   https://www.ncbi.nlm.nih.gov/pmc/articles/PMC3257651/.

45 Julian G. Martins, "EPA but Not DHA Appears to be Responsible for the Efficacy of Omega-3 Long Chain Polyunsaturated Fatty Acid Supplementation in Depression: Evidence from a Meta-Analysis of Randomized Controlled Trials," *Journal of the American College of Nutrition* 28, no. 5 (October 28, 2009): 525–42. doi:10.1080/07315724.2009.10719785. https://www.ncbi.nlm.nih.gov/pubmed/20439549.

46 Sheila M. Innis, "Dietary Omega 3 Fatty Acids and the Developing Brain," *Brain Research* 1237 (October 27, 2008): 35–43. doi:10.1016/j.brainres.2008.08.078.   https://www.ncbi.nlm.nih.gov/pubmed/18789910.

47 Meharban Singh, "Essential Fatty Acids, DHA and Human Brain," *Indian Journal of Pediatrics* 72 (March 2005): 239–42. https://www.ncbi.nlm.nih.gov/pubmed/15812120.

48 "Chapter 1: Key Elements of Healthy Eating Patterns," Key Recommendations: Components of Healthy Eating Patterns - 2015–2020 Dietary Guidelines. Health.gov. 2015. https://health.gov/dietaryguidelines/2015/guidelines/chapter-1/key-recommendations/.

49 "The Skinny on Fats," American Heart Association. https://www.heart.org/en/health-topics/cholesterol/prevention-and-

treatment-of-high-cholesterol-hyperlipidemia/the-skinny-on-fats.

50 "Omega-3 Fatty Acids Fact Sheet for Health Professionals," NIH Strengthening Knowledge and Understanding of Dietary Supplements. https://ods.od.nih.gov/factsheets/Omega3Fatty-Acids-HealthProfessional/.

51 "Dietary Proteins." U.S. National Library of Medicine. https://medlineplus.gov/dietaryproteins.html.

52 "Dietary Guidelines for Americans 2015–2020 8th Edition," Health.gov. 2015. https://health.gov/dietaryguidelines/2015/guidelines/.

53 Anika Knüppel, Martin J. Shipley, Clare H. Llewellyn, and Eric J. Brunner, "Sugar Intake from Sweet Food and Beverages, Common Mental Disorder and Depression: Prospective Findings from the Whitehall II Study," *Scientific Reports* 7, no. 1 (July 27, 2017). doi:10.1038/s41598-017-05649-7. https://www.ncbi.nlm.nih.gov/pmc/articles/PMC5532289/.

54 "Added Sugars," American Heart Association.Www.heart.org. https://www.heart.org/en/healthy-living/healthy-eating/eat-smart/sugar/added-sugars.

55 Starbucks Corporation. https://www.starbucks.ca/menu/nutrition-info.

56 "Caffeine: How Much Is Too Much?" Mayo Clinic, March 08, 2017. https://www.mayoclinic.org/healthy-lifestyle/nutrition-and-healthy-eating/in-depth/caffeine/art-20045678.

57 CDC - Data and Statistics - Sleep and Sleep Disorders. Centers for Disease Control and Prevention. https://www.cdc.gov/sleep/data_statistics.html.

58 "Melatonin: What You Need To Know," National Center for

Complementary and Integrative Health. https://nccih.nih.gov/health/melatonin.

59 "Serotonin," National Center for Biotechnology Information. https://www.ncbi.nlm.nih.gov/mesh/68012701.

60 "L-Tryptophan," MedlinePlus. https://medlineplus.gov/druginfo/natural/326.html.

61 Roseli Barbosa, Julieta Helena Scialfa, Ilza Mingarini Terra, José Cipolla-Neto, Valérie Simonneaux, and Solange Castro Afeche, "Tryptophan Hydroxylase Is Modulated by L-type Calcium Channels in the Rat Pineal Gland," *Life Sciences* 82, no. 9–10 (February 27, 2008): 529-35. doi:10.1016/j.lfs.2007.12.011. http://www.ncbi.nlm.nih.gov/pubmed/18221757.

62 "Vitamin B6 Fact Sheet for Health Professionals," NIH Strengthening Knowledge and Understanding of Dietary Supplements. https://ods.od.nih.gov/factsheets/VitaminB6-HealthProfessional/.

63 "Potassium," *Health Topics.* https://medlineplus.gov/potassium.html.

64 "Magnesium Fact Sheet for Health Professionals," NIH Strengthening Knowledge and Understanding of Dietary Supplements. https://ods.od.nih.gov/factsheets/Magnesium-HealthProfessional/.

65 "How Alcohol Affects the Quality–and Quantity–of Sleep," National Sleep Foundation. https://www.sleepfoundation.org/sleep-topics/how-alcohol-affects-sleep.

66 "Get the Facts: Drinking Water and Intake," Centers for Disease Control and Prevention. https://www.cdc.gov/nutrition/data-statistics/plain-water-the-healthier-choice.html.

67 *Dietary Reference Intakes: Water, Potassium, Sodium, Chloride,*

and Sulfate, February 11, 2004. http://www.nationalacademies.org/hmd/Reports/2004/Dietary-Reference-Intakes-Water-Potassium-Sodium-Chloride-and-Sulfate.aspx.

68 "Exercise and Stress: Get Moving to Manage Stress." Mayo Clinic, March 08, 2018. https://www.mayoclinic.org/healthy-lifestyle/stress-management/in-depth/exercise-and-stress/art-20044469.

69 https://adaa.org/understanding-anxiety/related-illnesses/other-related-conditions/stress/physical-activity-reduces-st.

70 *Sunscreen: How to Help Protect Your Skin from the Sun,* FDA.gov. https://www.fda.gov/drugs/understanding-over-counter-medicines/sunscreen-how-help-protect-your-skin-sun.